Stacking the coffins

Influenza, war and revolution in Ireland, 1918–19

IDA MILNE

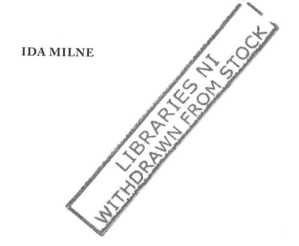
Manchester University Press

Published by Manchester University Press
Altrincham Street, Manchester M1 7JA
www.manchesteruniversitypress.co.uk

British Library Cataloguing-in-Publication Data
A catalogue record for this book is available from the British Library

ISBN 978 1 5261 2269 8 hardback

First published 2018

Typeset by Out of House Publishing
Printed in Great Britain
by CPI Group (UK) Ltd, Croydon, CR0 4YY

Contents

Figures and tables

Figures

Tables

Acknowledgements

This book has been a long time in genesis, and I have encountered many helpful hands along the way. I first wrote about the 1918–19 influenza pandemic for an MA dissertation in Maynooth in 2005, and fell in love with what was a promising but then under mined topic. David Lederer, Jackie Hill, Marian Lyons and Ray Gillespie were particularly helpful, and I am indebted to Jacinta Prunty for the firm grounding in statistics she gave her MA students. In 2006, I had the good fortune to have David Dickson agree to supervise me on the PhD programme at Trinity College, Dublin and am much indebted to him, particularly for encouraging me to find my own feet, the best skill a mentor can develop. My thesis examiners John Horne and Laurence Geary were thorough, supportive and gave appreciated advice. In TCD Department of History, there was a richly collegial community of postgraduates and postdoctoral fellows, encouraged by the then head of school, Jane Ohlmeyer. Elaine Murphy, Annaleigh Margey, Ann Downey, Frank Rynne, Kevin O'Sullivan, Eamon Darcy, Ciaran Wallace, Lisa-Marie Griffith, Eve Morrison, Justin Dolan Stover, Sean Lucey, Juliana Adelman, Justyna Pyz and Mary Muldowney all contributed to this work. The library and history administration staffs were most helpful. Ann Dolan, Joseph Clarke and Eunan O'Halpin were generous with ideas. Peter Rigney opened the railways archive on a bitterly cold winter's day in the arctic winter of 2010, and brought hot chocolate to keep fingers and brain working. Medical statistician Anthony Kinsella of the Royal College of Surgeons in Ireland was a good guide. Frank Bouchier Hayes has given me many leads, including directing me to the influenza cartoons in the British Cartoon Archive. My colleagues in the Department of History and Anthropology in Queen's University have also helped, particularly Marie Coleman, Elaine Farrell, Crawford Gribben, Fearghal McGarry, Olwen Purdue, Sean O'Connell and the late Keith Jeffery. In our working lives, we are supported by highly skilled office staff who do the horrible things we historians find complex and calm our troubled waters: my thanks to the History departmental staffs of Trinity

College Dublin, Queen's University Belfast and to Ann Donoghue and Catherine Heslin of Maynooth University. Colleagues from the Oral History Network of Ireland, the Oral History Society and the Oral History Association were most helpful. Catherine O'Connor of the University of Limerick has been a great friend and sounding board on many areas of scholarship, including oral history. I would not be on this path without the mentorship of Deirdre MacMahon and Maura Cronin. I am indebted to my dear friends in the social history of medicine for their scholarship and companionship: Jean Walker, Ian Miller, Clara Cullen, Ann Mc Lellan, Phil Gorey, Sean Lucey and the late Margaret Ó hÓgartaigh. Greta Jones, whose scholarship on disease history in Ireland is without peer, has been unstinting with her assistance. Patricia Marsh and I journeyed through our parallel PhD paths and subsequent research in a spirit of mutual support and development of our subject area, enjoying each other's achievements. Other colleagues at the Centres for the History of Medicine in Ulster and Dublin have added to this work. Guy Beiner, Barry Doyle, Virginia Crossman, William Murphy, Maurice Walsh, Ciara Breathnach, Ian d'Alton, Sean Farrell, Michael Laffan, Emmet O'Connor and Cormac Ó Gráda generously shared their work or advice with me. Breda Lavery, Keir Waddington and Ron Doel patiently read and suggested many improvements. Many medics have helped, including Yvonne O'Sullivan, Michelle Griffin and James Walsh.

I am grateful to Thomas Dark and the staff of Manchester University Press, and the encouraging words and useful advice of the anonymous readers.

Thanks also to Robert Mills and Harriet Wheelock of the Royal College of Physicians' heritage centre, Mary O'Doherty, archivist of the Royal College of Surgeons, Darragh O'Donoghue, archivist of the Allen Library, Margaret Doyle and Declan O'Keeffe of Clongowes Wood College, the staffs of the Wellcome Library, National Library of Ireland, General Register Office, National Archives of Ireland, National Archives, Kew, Dublin City Archives, Russell and John Paul II libraries in Maynooth, TCD libraries, QUB libraries, UCD libraries, Public Record Office of Northern Ireland in Belfast, Catholic Archdiocese of Dublin archive, Imperial War Museum in London, and county library services throughout Leinster, in particular Mario Corrigan in the local history office of Kildare library service; Cecile Chemin, former archivist for the Kildare, Meath and Wicklow county archives and Hazel Percival of Wexford library service. Local historians have engaged with what is in many ways a community project: I mention in particular Michael Dwyer, John Nangle, Willie Willoughby and members of the North Wexford Historical Society; Frank Taaffe; Catherine Boylan and members of Celbridge Historical Society; Liam Kenny; Ardclough History Group; the Uí Cinsealaigh

Society; Carlow Historical Society and Maynooth College Association of Local History.

Many other colleagues and friends have helped and better still encouraged along the way. Thanks to those unnamed – you know who you are – and my extended and adopted family of Milnes, MacMahons, Corrys, Deacons, James, Hattons, Tubridys, Elmes, Dooleys, my mother Sheila Milne, Eoghan Corry, and my inspiring daughters Síofra Milne Corry and Constance Corry.

The biggest debt of gratitude must go to the interviewees (and their families and carers) who generously opened their memories, their hearts and their thoughts to someone they barely knew, to enable a greater understanding of this most fascinating of topics, and to a network of contacts working diligently to find suitable people to interview. Special thanks to Jim Tancred, whose people skills opened many doors. The list of interviewees, and the value of their contributions, extends far beyond the limited scope of this text.

I am grateful to the Irish Research Council and Marie Curie Actions for the Elevate fellowship funding I received from 2014–18, and to the history departments at Maynooth University and Queen's University Belfast for hosting this fellowship.

This list is by no means complete. To those I have omitted, or who did not wish their names to be mentioned, your help was appreciated. None of the above are in any way to blame for flaws in what follows.

List of abbreviations

BOG	Board of Guardians
DMP	Dublin Metropolitan Police
GPB	General Prisons Board
GSWR	Great Southern and Western Railway
ICD	The International List of Classification of Death
JP	Justice of Peace
LGB	Local Government Board
MOH	Medical Officer of Health
MP	Member of (Westminster) Parliament
RAMI	Royal Academy of Medicine in Ireland
RG	Registrar General
SARS	Severe acute respiratory syndrome (coronavirus)
UDC	Urban District Council
WHO	World Health Organization
WNHA	Women's National Health Association

1

A 'mysterious malady' – or a 'perfect storm'?

When a major new epidemic of disease emerged in the ember days of the First World War, newspapers flagged it as a 'mystery disease', a 'mysterious malady'. It was not unexpected: recent wars had brought disease to civilian populations. Ironically, the disease that emerged was believed at first to have come from Spain – a country not involved in the war – and was thus named 'Spanish' influenza. The illness of the King of Spain and several thousand of his courtiers was widely reported in the newspapers, although by the time it infected the thirty-one-year-old Alfonso XIII, the French, US, British and German armies had already been depleted by influenza. Wartime censorship prevented these stories from appearing in newsprint, as neither side wanted to alert the other to its weakness.

The pandemic severely disrupted the work of the Paris Peace Conference, which was held to negotiate a lasting peace, as delegation after delegation fell prey to influenza over several months, including the three leaders, David Lloyd George, Georges Clemenceau and Woodrow Wilson. It is too taxing a challenge even to the playground of imagination to speculate what might have happened to the Anglo-Irish Treaty and the subsequent shape of Irish independence had Lloyd George succumbed to influenza in September 1918, when he fell ill while on a visit to Manchester; he came close to dying, and was still debilitated when he travelled to Paris for the negotiations. Woodrow Wilson spent a long time confined to quarters with the illness in the spring of 1919, inaccessible to all except his closest aides. Some believe that influenza made him paranoid for a time.

Statisticians and epidemiologists have, over time, variously estimated its death toll at between 20 million and 100 million people, with estimates for the number of people it infected now varying from one fifth to one half of the world's population. Most authorities now agree that it killed at least 40 million people.[1] Death registration was still rudimentary in many parts of the world, notably Africa, and therefore a more precise figure will never be known. It persuaded international health authorities to set up the influenza-monitoring systems that are still in use today.

As was the case for its putative parent organism, the war, Spanish influenza engenders heroic epithets. Variously described as 'the greatest disease the world has ever known', 'a greater killer than the Great War' or 'a greater killer than World Wars I and II combined', it is frequently added to the list of the other two most traumatic epidemic diseases the world's human population has experienced, namely the plagues of Justinian and the Black Death. This romanticisation of the pandemic (together with the recounting of particularly traumatic deaths, the dead lovers and the children found clinging to life in the arms of parents whose bodies were rigid in death) is perhaps associated with the social construct of the First World War. People writing about the social effects of the war tend to use a romantic and hyperbolic social construct befitting 'the war to end all wars', which was fought for 'the freedom of small nations'.

The Ireland of 1918 into which this disease arrived was going through an extraordinary period of rapid and often traumatic societal and political change. Many Irish were fighting in the First World War, from a multiplicity of motivations – Redmondites defending the 'freedom of small nations' having assumed a reward of home rule, loyalists protecting Empire, doctors and nurses dedicated to helping the suffering, adventurers seeking excitement, or people who saw it as a means of supporting their families. War was not only in the battlefields of Flanders or the Somme: it was evident on the newsstands, in the streets as soldiers come home on leave or in civilian hospital wards reserved for wounded soldiers, in the letters home from the front, or among the groups of women knitting socks and making comfort packages and bandages or raising funds for the Red Cross as acts of care for their absent loved ones. German U-boat activity in the Irish Sea and off the south and north coasts ramped up in 1917 and 1918, bringing the war more intensively to Irish waters.[2] The island's strategic location on a 'shipping superhighway' between Europe and North America made its waters a particular hunting ground. All vessels were threatened: troop carriers, passenger and merchant ships – targeted because of their cargoes of coal, food and other commodities – and even small fishing boats. Shortly after the United States entered the war in April 1917, US Navy destroyers were sent to Queenstown (now named Cobh) to escort shipping convoys, and the United States also established naval air stations at Wexford, Whiddy and Lough Foyle to help secure the Atlantic shipping lanes.

The war also increased dangers to – and fears about dangers to – public health. Both in Great Britain and in Ireland there was an awareness that infectious diseases such as smallpox, typhus and dysentery had a history of spreading to civilian populations from war zones.[3] Then there was the economic impact of the war, as inflation hit. The increased costs of food staples, such as bread, milk and eggs, allied with a severe scarcity of coal led to an apprehension that the resistance of the urban poor, in particular, to disease would be weakened. This issue was often discussed in the newspapers; the Dublin Castle administration and local authorities acted to control the price of essential commodities and to provide coal for the most vulnerable in order to increase the physical defences of the urban poor to disease. The parallel thread of the rising nationalism had been reinvigorated by the 'heroic' failure of the 1916 rebellion. The possible imposition of conscription was a contentious issue meeting with resistance from a broad spectrum of nationalist interests. Elections were about to be held in December 1918 for Ireland's representation at the British Parliament, but many of the Sinn Féin electoral candidates remained interned in Britain under a false pretext. The implementation of the Home Rule Act of 1914 had been suspended until after the war, but the goal of home rule was to be superseded by Sinn Féin's demand for a republic. Ireland was about to launch into the War of Independence and the Civil War, and attain self-government.

The pandemic represents a curious lacuna in Irish history, for it was omitted from the historiography until the last decade despite contemporary newspapers documenting its arrival and passage. The *Irish Times* and the *Irish Independent* in Dublin each carried perhaps twenty column inches a day on the second outbreak over a five-week period in October and November 1918, and again during the peak weeks of the third wave in March and April 1919. Vying with other important stories for space in the tiny newspapers of wartime, it often became the lead. Regional newspapers paid close attention to its progress, casting a wider than usual net to record stories of diamond production in the Transvaal being halted because so many of the staff were ill, or what European cities it was currently infecting. When it had passed, statisticians calculated that it was directly responsible for the deaths of 20,057 Irish – a figure that the Registrar General (RG) Sir William Thompson admitted was conservative. The medical professions and public health analysts also examined it using the methods of their own disciplines. Historians at best gave it a passing mention until this decade, even though Thompson had described it in the immediate aftermath as the greatest disease event since the Great Famine with its associated fevers and cholera, and the numbers of dead are on a scale comparable to the cholera epidemics of the nineteenth century. The cholera epidemics and the Great Famine have been popular themes for historians.

Another key factor in this failure to adequately record was that this new influenza was just one more disease of many that killed, year in, year out. While it looks striking from our modern lens because it killed young children and more surprisingly young adults, people not normally felled by seasonal influenza or other infectious diseases, death from infectious disease was a norm in this society. About 70,000 people died on the island each year, roughly double the number of annual deaths in the twenty-first century. One fifth of the annual deaths in the 1900s and 1910s were of children under five. Many died from wasting diseases of poverty, and from measles, scarlet fever, whooping cough, bronchitis and tuberculosis. Cramped substandard living accommodation for the poor elevated death levels in Ireland's cities, as in urban communities elsewhere. Dublin, with one third of its population living in tenements, had notorious health problems, although in the latter years of the 1910s the signs of change were promising as death rates beginning to fall. It was, in a way, hardly to be expected that one more disease, and at that a disease which re-emerged each year as a seasonal illness, should excite the attention of historians who were busy with their pens on other more pressing issues.

Nor was the omission by historians to record the pandemic surprising in a Europe laid waste by perhaps the most devastating war it had ever known. There were other things to record, even if the failure of trains to run, factories to operate or crops to be saved because of lack of manpower caused by this illness might have been deemed significant enough to record had it been ascribed to a different cause. And there were failures to assess the effects of the pandemic by historians in countries with no other distractions.

For forgetting the flu was not an Irish phenomenon: it was a universal one. This curious gap in history is truly surprising when one considers the ability of influenza to permeate every layer of society, every organisation and social structure. It affected everything. The Spanish influenza pandemic silenced whole communities as it passed through, extracting a devastating death toll and even more astounding numbers of sufferers. At a micro level, families were flattened, incapable of doing anything except struggling to live; often they failed in that struggle in a most dramatic manner, presenting a pathetic tableau to would-be rescuers who broke down doors to find entire families either dead or beyond help, and sometimes dying together in the same bed. At a macro level, the disease paralysed the war and sectors of commerce and industry, and disrupted stock markets.

In the immediate aftermath of the pandemic, most of the literature about the flu was of a medical or statistical nature. There followed a long interval when little was written about it. Since the 1970s the literature slowly started to build. By the 1990s, the literature on Spanish influenza was burgeoning. It was influenced by three factors: new scientific methods which enabled the recovery of previously inaccessible evidence; increased attention from historians (in Ireland partly influenced by a new openness to discussion of Irish involvement in the First World War); and popular interest as world health authorities warned that a new pandemic of influenza was overdue. Pandemics are understood to run at intervals of roughly thirty years, and the last one had been in 1968, in a world recently threatened with the possible escalation of severe acute respiratory syndrome (SARS) and H5N1 avian influenza into significant epidemics. This popular interest surged in 2009, as a new strain of influenza caused an epidemic with alarming morbidity and mortality in Mexico, which some thought comparable with the 1918–19 pandemic. The strain was renamed Influenza A 2009 H1N1 by the World Health Organization and was officially declared a pandemic when it met certain criteria, but turned out to be something of a false alarm, perhaps, as some authorities suggest, because of the success of mass vaccination programmes.[4]

What did experts know?

In an Irish context, both physicians and statisticians conducted the analysis in the immediate aftermath. The *Dublin Journal of Medical Science* carried papers written by Captain John Speares and Dr George Peacocke and others about the aetiology of the disease, and methods they had used to treat it.[5] The RG Sir William Thompson focused on it in his annual returns and in the *Dublin Journal of Medical Science* and the *Journal of the Statistical and Social Inquiry Society of Ireland*.[6]

There were two major international works written in the immediate aftermath which are frequently quoted even at a remove of ninety years, as authoritative works on aspects of the pandemic. The first was a series of essays on the pandemic by experts from different medical disciplines, which was edited by F.G. Crookshank and published in London in 1922.[7] In an exploration of knowledge about influenza through the ages, he advocated that the 'pitch of confusion and degree of failure' surrounding the diagnosis of influenza in the Spanish flu epidemic might be explained by looking at the incidence of influenza-type illnesses in the preceding years:

> In 1915–16 a prevalence of 'grip' of such magnitude as to have been called pandemic swept through the United States … accompanied by outbreaks of pneumonia and by an epidemic in New York which was called poliomyelitis although pathologically of the nature of meningo-encephalomyelitis. The health authorities decided that this 'grip', because it was not associated with Pfeiffer's bacillus, was only a pseudo-influenza. The epidemiological liaison between the 'Grip', the pneumonia, and the poliomyelitis was completely missed, and in many cases of … encephalitis lethargica were on the Pacific coast diagnosed as botulism, and ascribed, in the most light hearted fashion, to the consumption of canned beans and tomatoes.[8]

In an essay on the different presentations of influenza, W.H. Hamer made a point pertinent to the calculation of statistics about the 1918–19 pandemic – that influenza is typically misdiagnosed unless there is known evidence of an epidemic. He suggested that many cases of influenza during the war were misdiagnosed as dengue, trench fever, pyrexia or fever of unknown origin (known as PUO), or disordered action of the heart, a common sequel of influenza. He also pointed out that illnesses resembling the Spanish flu were prevalent in London and other places from 1915. Hamer said that one thing was certain: more ought to be known about influenza if the progress of civilisation were not to be seriously impeded. He said: 'A philosopher's stone is needed which will transmute influenza, when it threatens prevalence in pandemic phase, at any rate into a common cold, if it be not possible to render it entirely innocuous.'[9]

During the winters of 1915 and 1916, physicians at the Aldershot Command reported an unusual influenza-type illness, which sometimes manifested in a heliotrope cyanosis (later to become a signature feature of the Spanish flu). Adolphe Abrahams reported their findings in his essay, saying that the illness was very distressing as it had a very high mortality rate and there was no effective treatment. At the time, physicians in the Aldershot Command believed that the influenza-type illness there was peculiar to the Aldershot Command area, which had a reputation for the presentation of anomalous respiratory diseases. But it soon became apparent that a similar disease was occurring in other places, when Hammond, Rolland and Shore published an article entitled 'Purulent Bronchitis', which was based on their observation of cases occurring in France; the publication of this and the Aldershot findings were swiftly followed by reports of similar groups of cases from many parts of Europe. Thus, in Crookshank's work the evidence of three essayists suggests that a form of Spanish flu was circulating in Britain and in France since 1915, but diagnosed as purulent bronchitis.[10] This is significant, as others have claimed in more recent years that the disease had its origins in America in 1918 and was brought eastwards to the battlefields rather than beginning earlier in Europe.

Crookshank also observed that the great pandemics of influenza were not isolated phenomena, but were each part of a series of organised disturbances of health spread over an influenzal period, lasting roughly for the whole world some five years or so, with central waves of influenza within that period. He stressed the importance of studying the precursors of what he called 'picaresque catastrophes'. His words may have implications for the world of the early twenty-first century with its outbreaks of Middle Eastern respiratory syndrome (MERS), severe acute respiratory syndrome (SARS), H5N1 avian influenza and, more recently, the 2009 H1N1 strain of influenza.

The second, written by the bacteriologist Edwin Oakes Jordan and published in 1927, was significant because Jordan estimated world mortality in the pandemic at over 21.6 million people. This figure proved that the pandemic had killed more people than the First World War, which overshadowed it in terms of tragedy and public awareness.[11] Jordan's estimate has since undergone a series of revisions.[12]

For the ensuing fifty years, most of the works dealing with the influenza pandemic were either memoirs or novels. Among the best known of these would be Katharine Anne Porter's novel *Pale Horse, Pale Rider* (1939). Porter's story follows Miranda, a young woman working for a newspaper in Denver in 1918, as the world war continued to influence people's lives. As funeral processions for flu victims pass regularly through the streets, one of the characters relates a story to Miranda that encapsulates the myths that surrounded the flu: 'They say that it is really caused by germs brought by a German ship to Boston. Somebody reported seeing a strange, thick, greasy-looking cloud float up out of Boston Harbour.' Robert Graves related in his autobiography his determination to return home to his family in England after catching the flu while stationed with the third battalion of the Royal Welch in Limerick. His demobilisation papers were not complete on 13 February, with demobilisation due to be halted the following day. He tricked a superior officer into signing them and bolted for home without the necessary secret demobilisation code-marks, fearing the effects that suffering the influenza in an Irish military hospital would have on his war-damaged lungs. By chance, he shared a taxi from Fishguard to Waterloo with the Cork district demobilisation officer, who gave him the code-marks. By the time he reached his home at Hove, he had septic pneumonia, and was not expected to live. However, he determined not to succumb to Spanish influenza, after having survived the war. The disease had already killed his mother-in-law.[13]

Interest rekindled

Apart from the occasional reference in a memoir or novel there was little further work done on the pandemic until the 1970s, when Alfred Crosby and Richard Collier rekindled interest in the issue. Collier collected contemporary letters, specially written accounts and interviews with 1,708 survivors of the pandemic in Europe, North and South America, Australia and New Zealand, Africa, India and Borneo. Collier's collection of testimonies has merit in its own right as a collection of historical evidence but it offers no analysis of the flu's impact or why it was forgotten.

Alfred Crosby's *America's Forgotten Pandemic*, first published in 1976, is regarded as a definitive account of the pandemic in the United States of America, and is constantly used as a reference by other influenza historians. It systematically covers the effects of influenza in major US cities, territories and among the US armed forces. Some credit him with the rekindling of academic interest in the topic. His chronicling of influenza illness among the American delegation at the Paris Peace Conference gives a good insight into the way in which influenza upset the talks. Colonel House, Woodrow Wilson's chief advisor on foreign affairs, was disabled by it for the last few weeks of 1918 and the early weeks of 1919. Other members of the delegation were also ill with the flu at this time, and Willard Straight died on 1 December 1918. House himself believed his mental agility was weakened in the aftermath of the attack. By early spring, in one of the peak weeks for influenza in Paris, doctors paid 125 house calls in one day to the members of the American delegation ill with the flu. On 3 April, President Wilson caught flu. Crosby asked how Wilson – determined prophet of 'peace without victory' – could compromise his principles to agree to the Treaty of Versailles in the days after the influenza attack; he notes that a number of people in close contact with the president in the nego-tiations felt that his grasp of issues was severely affected by the dis-ease. The President seemed to become paranoid for a time, perhaps as a consequence of the influenza attack. Crosby also drew attention to the forgetting of the flu:

> The most important and almost incomprehensible fact about the Spanish flu is that it killed millions upon millions of people in a year or less. Nothing else – no infection, no war, no famine – has ever killed so many in such a short period. And yet it has never inspired awe, not in 1918 and not since, not among the citizens of any particular land and not among the citizens of the United States.[14]

Given Ireland's strategic significance for the US Navy convoy escorts and airbases, Crosby's discussion of flu in the navy is particularly relevant here. Forty per cent of the US Navy caught influenza in 1918. Close quarters and overcrowding on board ships offered ideal conditions for spreading influenza; despite repeated requests by

US naval medical staff, no effort was made to make the conditions onboard less conducive to the spread of the disease until October 1918, as the evidence proved that shipping soldiers in such unhealthy conditions was counterproductive. Crosby said that 4,136 officers and men died from influenza, twice as many as to enemy action, despite 'the best efforts of Germany's undersea fleet'. He noted that although the situation was bad among navy personnel with a case fatality rate of 1.5 per cent, soldiers on the troop ships they shepherded across the Atlantic had a much higher rate of death, at 6.43 per cent.[15] The then assistant secretary of the US Navy Franklin Delano Roosevelt returned home from the Paris Peace Conference on the grim *Leviathan*, a troop carrier on which many died, with influenza which had turned into double pneumonia, but survived to become president of his country.

Eighty years on, the literature burgeons

By the 1990s, literature about the disease had burgeoned, through the increased interest from historians, scientists such as John Oxford and Jeffery Taubenberger, who were using new scientific methods to collect new evidence, and by national and world health authorities increasingly concerned about the threat of the development of a new influenza virus with pandemic capabilities.

As public awareness about the pandemic increases, so too do the potential book sales, and there are a number of works that have tried to capitalise on this growing public awareness. In this genre of popular accounts of disease stories, perhaps Gina Kolata's *Flu* is the most impressive. Kolata's best-selling book serves a useful role in tracking the scientific exploration into the Spanish flu pandemic in the late twentieth century, and provides colourful insights into the human dynamic behind such exploration.[16] One division of the American Army, the eighty-eighth, arrived in France on 17 September 1918, and fought on the front lines from 26 October until the end of the war on 11 November, lost 444 men to influenza and only had ninety killed, wounded, missing or captured in war.[17] Yet even biographers of what Kolata calls 'the great men of American medicine' involved in ensuring the health of the US Army during the war barely mention the disease.

Phillips and Killingray

In 1998, a conference held at the University of Cape Town drew together influenza historians from all over the world. The disciplinary perspectives were broad, and included virology, pathology, epidemiology, demography, history, anthropology, geography and gender studies. Sixteen of the thirty-six contributors to the conference wrote articles in the Society for the Social History of Medicine (SSHM) series' *The Spanish Influenza Pandemic of 1918–1919: New Perspectives* (2003), edited by Howard Phillips and David Killingray, which is perhaps the most comprehensive text on the pandemic since the publication of Crookshank's essays on influenza in 1922.[18] As few scholarly attempts have been made to examine the calamity in its many-sided complexity, this work began the process on a global multidisciplinary scale, seeking to apply the insights of a wide range of social and medical sciences to an investigation of the pandemic. Topics covered include the historiography of the pandemic, its virology, the enormous demographic impact, the medical and governmental responses it elicited, and its long-term effect, particularly the recent attempts to identify the precise causative virus from specimens taken from the flu victims in 1918, or victims buried in the arctic permafrost. The contributors include many names familiar to anyone who has read about the flu pandemic: John Oxford, Edwin D. Kilbourne, Jürgen Müller, Geoffrey Rice, D. Ann Herring, Niall Johnson, Jeffery Taubenberger and Beatriz Echeverri. The editors also have solid credentials as flu historians. Howard Phillips published his doctoral thesis on the impact of Spanish influenza pandemic on South Africa in 1990, and David Killingray has done work on the impact of influenza on the British Empire.

In the foreword, the virologist John Oxford wrote that he viewed 1918 as a pivotal year in human history: 'Contiguous with the end of the Great War came the huge surge of global influenza. As soldiers filled liners and cargo ships to return home, as they thought to safety, in Australia, South Africa, New Zealand and the United States, they were looking forward to family reunion parties, village gatherings and victory marches …'. Probably, he said, never before or since have so many young people travelled together in such overcrowded circumstances. 'From the point of view of a miniscule virus spread from person to person in droplets from coughs, this was an unprecedented and gloriously unique opportunity – influenza took it ... so the northern autumn of 1918 witnessed a singular and cataclysmic event.'[19]

Oxford observed that there must have been many more acts of heroism in homes of the world in the great pandemic than in the First World War as husbands and wives and families strained to cope with the diseased, and as many families died together. Nevertheless, most sufferers survived: 95 per cent of the world's population survived the pandemic, including Oxford's own father. Oxford noted that in the preceding ten years scientists using modern technology have been able to pursue the genetic structure of the virus, spurring virological interest in the pandemic.

> As a virologist I would want to know where the virus came from. Even as the conference was proceeding in Cape Town my students had uncovered a description of an earlier outbreak at Étaples in northern France in the winter of 1916 ... I can think of no more likely spot for a virus to mutate and spread. We may have to rename the virus the French influenza rather that the Spanish influenza, and to ascribe the date to 1916 rather than to 1918, but there is no disputing two things. First, 1918 saw a wave of infection and respiratory death that no one on the planet would want to live through again, and second, as virologists, we do expect another influenza pandemic to visit and in our most pessimistic moments wonder whether, in spite of new anti-neuraminidase inhibitors, amantadine and influenza vaccines, we will eventually experience a 1918 scenario of our own.

The SSHM series published Niall Johnson's *Britain and the 1918–19 Influenza Pandemic: a Dark Epilogue* in 2006. It is a brave and energetic attempt to write a 'total' history, examining the environmental, geographical, political, cultural, biological and medical aspects of the pandemic in Britain, and using multiple sources, approaches and gazes to do so.[20] He discussed the history and aetiology of influenza, and the pandemic geography of the 1918–19 attack, using maps to illustrate the wave pattern.[21] Mark Honigsbaum's *Living with Enza* is based on previously unpublished and mostly British testimonies from Collier's interview collection, now housed in the Imperial War Museum. His work is essentially a popular discourse using the Collier collection and other memoirs as primary sources, reworking some concepts about Spanish influenza that have already been developed in other work.[22]

The availability of high-quality statistical data on health in Norway and Sweden during the period 1918–20 (some areas of Scandinavia suffered a fourth wave in 1920) has provided an exciting basis for social studies of the disease in these countries, at a level which is not possible in most other countries, including Ireland and Great Britain. I draw attention to a couple here as examples. Elisabeth Engberg's studies of Spanish influenza have looked at social and official responses to the pandemic in rural communities in northern Sweden, a departure from the normal convention of looking at influenza in urban communities. In the five studied rural communities, the official response was sparse and reactive, and the presence of pandemic influenza is almost invisible in the municipal records. Potentially preventive measures, such as school closures and bans on public gatherings, were not used. Engberg comments on the local authorities' apparent inertia during the Spanish influenza, and on other issues – the struggle with wartime hardship, food crisis and a strained economy, an insufficient public health administration, a national preventive policy primarily aimed at the prevention of cholera, and the continued use of traditional methods to deal with crises in society.[23] Svenn-Erik Mamelund's work on Spanish influenza in Norway has challenged the commonly held perspective that this influenza was a socially neutral disease as far as mortality was concerned. He suggested that this perspective gained credence because media outlets and academic and popular accounts have tended to emphasise the high-profile victims, among them Alfonso XIII of Spain, the world leaders at the Parish Peace Conference, the Norwegian painter Edvard Munch, who all survived, and members of the royal families of Sweden and Britain, who did not. Mamelund's study combined multivariate event history analysis with individual and household-level data to test this perspective. He found that the size of accommodation, which was a perfect proxy for rent and therefore probably also for income, was negatively and significantly associated with mortality. The wealthy and highly educated probably had lower mortality from influenza and pneumonia than the poor and less educated because the former benefited from earlier (self) diagnosis, bed rest and nursing (paid for by saved capital and health insurance, which enabled them to be away from work), fewer pre-existing lung (tuberculosis) or heart diseases, and few or no nutritional problems.[24]

While the Irish literature on the pandemic as a rule follows the pattern of the international literature, it deviated from that pattern in the last thirty years. The international literature has gathered pace since Crosby's and Collier's works, but nothing emerged from Irish historians. Within the past ten years, work has been amassing on the Irish experience of the pandemic from three PhD dissertations, of which Caitríona Foley's *The Last Irish Plague* was the first published monograph, and this is the second.[25] Patricia Marsh who researched the Ulster experience and this author have both published chapters on the influenza pandemic in edited collections, and have co-written an article on it in *History Ireland* with Guy Beiner.[26] Two television documentaries have been made about the Irish experience of the pandemic: *Aicid*, an Irish-language production for TG4 by the independent production company Arkhive, and an episode of the RTE documentary series on disease, *Outbreak*; the author of this work was involved in both documentaries.[27]

This book describes how the 1918–19 influenza pandemic unfolded in an Irish context, during an extraordinary period when Irish society was experiencing the trauma of the war and the rapid move towards independence. The influenza pandemic made a substantive impact on both these areas. Robert A. Aronowitz has argued that studying the impact of a disease on society is a useful exercise for the historian as disease can often evoke and reflect collective responses, permitting an understanding of the values and attitudes of the society in which they occur.[28] What follows shows the aptness of his concept is in the context of the 1918–19 pandemic in the maelstrom society of a revolutionary Ireland.

The outbreak of influenza seemed to fester every sore, exacerbating already difficult relationships or situations. Chapter 2 relates the story of the disease as it is interpreted by journalists, showing how they narrated its arrival and progress, and how certain themes emerged through that narration. Influenza emerges from the war conditions, whether in Europe or in America (see Chapter 5), but as a news story it competes with war for primacy. If Irish society was a simmering pot in 1918, the outbreak of influenza was the heat that helped it to bubble over. It became part of every facet of Irish society, from the private lives of families to trade, the war and the conscription crisis, the defence of Irish waters by the US and British navies, the growing disaffection with Dublin Castle administration and corresponding strengthening confidence of the national movement, and the need to reform a faltering health system. Statistics hold the key to understanding which age groups, classes, employments and regions suffered the most death; this topic is explored in Chapter 3. The pandemic killed at a conservative estimate 23,000 Irish people when excess pneumonia cases are included. It probably infected about 800,000 more, or about one fifth of the island's 1911 population. This book looks at how the influenza pandemic overburdened the Poor Law dispensary service (Chapter 4) and the hospitals (Chapter 6) and in doing so highlights not only the impact the world war was having on Irish medical provision, but the gross inadequacy of the system itself. The system had long been recognised to be in need of reform: the influenza pandemic helped to inform the decisions of the Public Health Council, which made radical recommendations on healthcare reforms in 1919, just months after the pandemic had abated in Ireland. The pandemic exacerbated political tensions both between the increasingly nationalist BOGs who administered the Poor Law at a local level and the Local Government Board for Ireland, and between nationalists and the Dublin Castle administration. In a curious coincidence of history, the pandemic in Ireland ran parallel with the so-called 'German' plot (Chapter 8). This was a scheme devised by the administration to intern leading anti-conscription campaigners, as the administration, which was led by newly appointed Lord Lieutenant Sir John French, sought to impose conscription in Ireland in 1918. It became part of the Sinn Féin propaganda machine, as it killed two of the internees, one in the run-up to the pivotal general election of December 1918. It appeared to confirm nationalist warnings that internment would pose health risks to the detained, although the real story is more complex. The book also looks at contemporary medical understanding of the disease, and how it punctured the new-found confidence of the medical profession in bacteriology, as they failed to find an effective treatment (Chapter 5). Chapter 9 explores the long-term impacts of influenza pandemic.

Most poignantly, Chapter 7 unveils the patient experience of disease through a series of oral history interviews the author carried out with survivors or with the families of people who died in the pandemic. These interviews reveal how families sometimes lost several members, and economic circumstances were often changed by the loss of one or both parents. They also tell the story of small children who survived against the odds, and lived well into their nineties or hundreds to tell the tale.

Notes

1 E.O. Jordan, *Epidemic Influenza: a Survey* (Chicago, IL: AMA, 1927), p. 229. Edwin Oakes Jordan first estimated the mortality from Spanish influenza as 21.6 million people in 1926. The World Health Organization currently estimates that the pandemic killed between 40 and 50 million. There were two subsequent influenza pandemics in the twentieth century, the Asian pandemic in 1957 killed two million people and the Hong Kong pandemic in 1968–69, which killed one million people (Source: World Health Organization, www.who.int/csr/disease/influenza/pandemic10things/en/, accessed 5 October 2010).

2 Michael Kennedy, 'On the Atlantic frontline: Ireland's lightkeepers and lightshipmen and the outbreak of unrestricted submarine warfare'; paper presented at Winning the Western Approaches: Unrestricted Submarine Warfare and the US Navy in Ireland, 1917–18 conference, University College Cork, 6 July 2017.

3 For a useful discussion of this topic, see Hans Zinsser. *Rats, Lice and History* (Boston, MA: Little, Brown, 1935).

4 John Oxford, 'Epidemics past present and future', public lecture in the Paccar Theatre of the Science Gallery, Trinity College, Dublin, May 2010.

5 George Peacocke, 'Influenza', *Dublin Journal of Medical Science*, 3rd series, no. 146 (1918), pp. 249–53. John Speares, 'Influenza', *Dublin Journal of Medical Science*, 3rd series, no. 146 (1918), pp. 253–8.

6 William J. Thompson, 'Mortality from influenza in Ireland', *Journal of the Statistical and Social Inquiry Society of Ireland*, xiv, no. 1 (1919/1920), pp. 1–14. William J. Thompson, 'Mortality from influenza in Ireland', *Dublin Journal of Medical Science*, 4th series (1920), pp. 174–86.

7 F.G. Crookshank, ed., *Influenza: Essays by Several Authors* (London: Heineman, 1922). See Chapter 7 for a fuller description of encephalitis lethargica, a sleeping sickness often observed in connection with epidemic influenza.

8 Ibid., p. 33.

9 W.H. Hamer, 'The phases of influenza', in Crookshank, ed., *Influenza*, pp. 102–27.

10 Adolphe Abrahams, 'Influenza: some clinical and therapeutic considerations', in Crookshank, ed., *Influenza*, pp. 314–50. J.A.R. Hammond, W. Rolland and T.H.G. Shore, 'Purulent bronchitis', *Lancet*, ii (1917), p. 41.

11 Edwin O. Jordan, *Epidemic Influenza: a Survey* (Chicago, IL: American Medical Association, 1927).

12 Richard Collier, *The Plague of the Spanish Lady* (London: Atheneum, 1974).

13 Robert Graves, *Goodbye to All That* (rev. edn, London: Penguin, 1960), pp. 290–7.

14 Alfred W. Crosby, *America's Forgotten Pandemic: the Influenza of 1918* (Cambridge: Cambridge University Press, 2003), p. 311.
15 Ibid., pp. 122–3.
16 Gina Kolata, *Flu* (New York: Farrar, Straus and Giroux, 1999).
17 Kolata, *Flu*, p. 50.
18 Howard Phillips and David Killingray, eds, *The Spanish Influenza Pandemic of 1918–1919, New Perspectives* (Abingdon: Routledge, 2003).
19 Ibid., p. xvii.
20 Niall Johnson, *Britain and the 1918–19 Influenza Pandemic: a Dark Epilogue* (Abingdon: Routledge, 2006).
21 Ibid., p. 136.
22 Mark Honigsbaum, *Living with Enza* (Basingstoke: Palgrave, 2009).
23 Elisabeth Engberg, 'The invisible influenza: Community response to pandemic influenza in rural northern Sweden 1918–20', *Vária Historia*, xlii, no. 25 (2009), pp. 429–6.
24 Svenn-Erik Mamelund, 'A socially neutral disease? Individual social class, household wealth and mortality from Spanish influenza in two socially contrasting parishes in Kristiania 1918–19', *Social Science & Medicine*, lxii (2006), pp. 923–40.
25 Caitríona Foley, *The Last Irish Plague* (Dublin: Irish Academic Press, 2011).
26 Guy Beiner, Patricia Marsh and Ida Milne, 'Greatest killer of the twentieth century: the great flu in 1918–19, *History Ireland* (March–April 2009), pp. 40–3, republished in John Gibney, Tommy Graham and Georgina Laragy, eds, *History Ireland – 1916–18 Changed Utterly: Ireland after the Rising* (Dublin: Wordwell, 2017).
27 A selection of recent publications emerging from these three PhD studies include Beiner, Marsh and Milne, 'Greatest killer of the twentieth century: the great flu in 1918–19', pp. 40–3. Caitríona Foley, *The Last Irish Plague: the Great Flu in Ireland 1918–19* (Dublin: Irish Academic Press, 2011), Patricia Marsh, 'The war and influenza: the impact of the First World War on the 1918–19 influenza pandemic in Ulster', in Ian Miller and David Durnin, eds, *Medicine, Health and Irish Experiences of Conflict, 1914–45* (Manchester: Manchester University Press, 2016) and Ida Milne, 'Influenza: the Irish Local Government Board's last great crisis', in Virginia Crossman and Sean Lucey, eds, *Healthcare in Ireland and Britain 1850–1970: Voluntary, Regional and Comparative Perspectives.* (London: Institute for Historical Research, 2015), pp. 217–36.
28 Robert Aronowitz, 'Lyme disease: the social construction of a new disease and its social consequences', *Milbank Quarterly*, lxix, no. 1 (1991), pp. 79–112.

2

The flu: a news perspective

In the first six months of 1918, war dominated the news agenda, shifting between a focus on the major battles in Belgium and France, and the domestic impositions of war – inflation, Irish soldiers who died and the growing tensions over the threat of conscription in Ireland to provide army manpower, which was being energetically resisted by a broad spectrum of nationalist groups who were holding mass meetings around the country. Increased German U-boat activity in Irish waters also often featured in the news pages. Irish news was a complex network of threads in 1918. Into this web, in the early summer of 1918, came the largest infectious disease event in modern world history.

Newspapers document what was in the public domain about the influenza pandemic as it occurred. One can assess its day-to-day newsworthiness by the standard measure of news value, the number of newspaper column inches, observing its low-key arrival and then the waves and troughs in coverage as it worsens in communities, stilling daily routines as those infected take to their sickbed, and finally its passage. Newspaper coverage has enabled the identification of three waves of the disease, in the early summer and autumn of 1918, and in the spring of 1919; the RG's weekly death statistics only cover Dublin. One can see its pathway as it moves around from the ports – the points of entry – to cities and villages, through the pages of the national and regional newspapers. From newspapers, one can see what issues emerged from it and place it in the context of what other stories were making the news. This chapter aims to recreate the tensions about this new disease emerging in the final days of the war and particularly focuses on counties in Leinster – Dublin, Wicklow,

Wexford, Kilkenny, Kildare and Louth – as statistics show that the eastern province bore the brunt of the second and worst wave of the pandemic in Ireland.

In the early part of the twentieth century, the Irish news industry was thriving. Generally, each market town had at least one title, and sometimes more, reflecting the often different political allegiances of local populations. Provincial papers were usually published once a week; typically, during the 1910s, they carried not only local, but also international and war news, as it related to their population base. Cities like Belfast and Dublin had several daily morning and evening newspapers, again serving different population bases. The *Irish Times* was popular with those who worked in government and with an educated pro-establishment population, generally Unionist or urban Protestant. It had modest sales of about 30,000 copies a day.[1] The *Irish Independent* was the best-selling daily title at about 100,000 copies; it and the *Freeman's Journal* (also circa 30,000 daily sales) were popular across the religious divide, and the voices of moderate nationalism and of business. The *Evening Herald*, the leading Dublin-based evening paper, had a strong political focus and seemed more interested in stories about labouring classes. It covered mainly city and international news, but was also distributed to the provinces. Each of these papers took feeds from English press and from the wire services, such as Reuters and the American-based Associated Press, which gave them fast comprehensive access to international news.

The diverse strands of Irish life were fighting a tight daily battle for column inches in the newspapers, as war newspapers were very small owing to the scarcity of newsprint and to censorship. The *Irish Independent* had just six pages, usually with three covered in advertisements. News of the war generally won that battle, with as many details of war activities as were permitted by the war censors. Newspaper layout was rather different to that of today: the front page was covered in the more expensive advertisements, often advertising products related to the world war. As well as a daily digest of manoeuvres across Continental Europe, daily and regional weekly papers often carried a roll of honour of the Irish officers and rank-and-file men who were dead, missing, wounded, or 'in German hands'.

Apart from war news, other themes which predominated and interlinked in the complex web of Irish current affairs in 1918 were the threat of conscription and the 'German' plot. Prime Minister David Lloyd George's Military Service Act came into force on 18 April, leading to the withdrawal of the Irish Parliamentary Party from the House of Commons in protest at the proposed extension of conscription to Ireland, the first of a series of protests by Irish political groups.[2] In mid-May, about a hundred Sinn Féin and Volunteer leaders and others active in the anti-conscription movement were rounded up and interned in Ireland and Great Britain: an establishment effort to discredit them. The pretext was that a German agent had been arrested off the coast of Co. Clare having come to Ireland to plot an intrigue with Sinn Féin. The authorities had deluded themselves into believing that a smear on the Sinn Féin leadership would lead to the loss of public support from the middle ground. The detention without trial of these men and women, many of them prominent in Irish society, such as Countess Constance Markievicz and Maud Gonne McBride, as well as leading Sinn Féin politicians Arthur Griffith and Eamon de Valera, and some medical doctors, led to deep unrest among the populace. Even the archly conservative *Church of Ireland Gazette* called for an open trial of the internees, saying 'it is to be regretted that, with that lack of instinct for the right thing which seems again to be gathering about its dealings with Ireland, the Government has not taken this course'.[3] The plight of the internees was to become entangled with the influenza epidemic.

By early June, the Germans had reached the Marne, and were close to Paris; the war on the Continent was impinging more directly at home, as German submarine activity increased in the Irish Sea. The sinking of fishing boats from Kilkeel and Ardglass in Co. Down caused an outburst from the leader writer in the *Irish Independent* of Monday, 3 June 1918: 'They are not content with sinking Irish merchant and passenger steamers whenever they get the chance, but carry on their ruthless warfare against poor fishing folk.' Dublin, Arklow and south-coast fishermen had already been hit.[4] Lord Lieutenant Viscount John French issued a proclamation looking for 50,000 new Irish recruits by October.[5] Recruitment and conscription to provide human fodder for the hungry belly of war were constant themes in the news pages.

The first wave: a 'mysterious malady' in June 1918

By 10 June, a journalist at the *Belfast Newsletter* reported an unusual outbreak of illness in Belfast, mostly among soldiers and female factory workers. The somewhat self-contradictory headline 'An epidemic in Belfast – no cause for alarm' expressed much of the tension as people kept a watchful eye on illnesses developing during the war. Previous wars were associated with diseases moving into civilian populations. The conclusion of the 1870–71 Franco-Prussian War with a pandemic of smallpox was very much in the conscious memory of the public, the medical professions and the British Government; it was often alluded to in official reports and in the newspapers.[6] The *Newsletter* reporter described symptoms that were reassuringly influenza-like. Having interviewed a city doctor the previous evening to see what was happening, the journalist aimed to calm public fears about the nature of this illness, and confirmed that in the doctor's opinion the disease was nothing sinister, that the symptoms are mostly those of influenza, a usually manageable seasonal illness:

> Many exaggerated stories have been circulated in the city regarding the outbreak, but, as already stated, there is absolutely no cause for alarm upon the part of the public. In the cases investigated there is nothing in the nature of trench fever, cerebro-spinal meningitis, or the mysterious botulism.[7]

The epidemic continued to develop in east Ulster. On Thursday, 20 June, the *Irish Independent* reported 'Mysterious scourge is spreading':

> A virulently infectious disease resembling influenza in its symptoms has spread rapidly through Belfast. In many cases entire households have been seized, and in some industrial establishments entire departments have been obliged to close. About a dozen schools in the east of the city have been closed, as, although children suffer less than adults, they spread the infection, and probably all other schools will follow suit. Doctors recommend victims to take to bed as soon as signs appear and to remain there till the last traces go, as there have been cases of fatal relapses. A similar state of affairs is reported from Ballinasloe, where over 60 people have been prostrate. Sudden collapses are here the most striking feature, the disease giving no warning and the victim being struck down almost instantaneously. It is stated that influenza is just now rife in Berlin, and is spreading on the continent.[8]

This was the first announcement that the Dublin paper carried of the influenza pandemic that was to sweep across the world in three waves by the spring of the following year, killing at least 20 million and possibly many millions more. Once again, the story conveyed both the sense of alarm at the odd appearance of influenza out of season, and the author's judgement that alarm needed to be managed in order to prevent panic.

The provincial papers were also by then echoing this alarm at the outbreak in Belfast of what the *Midland Reporter and Westmeath Nationalist* called the 'mystery malady' or 'mysterious war disease.'[9] They reported that one firm, a munitions business, had been closed down and fumigated because of the malady; work was being suspended for the week owing to the illness of mostly women workers. An outbreak was also reported among soldiers in the city, and those suffering from the disease were isolated. No deaths had been reported.

As the war continued with news of the intense struggle for Venice, and for Rheims on the Western Front, the newspapers also tracked the influenza epidemic's progress. The leader writer in the *Irish Independent* on Monday 24 June explained that the epidemic was first reported from Spain, where the King and one third of his subjects were infected, and in various parts of England and Ireland:

> It is pretty virulent in London … as well as in a number of soldiers' camps. In Ireland it first appeared in Belfast, then in Ballinasloe, and now it is prevalent in Athlone and Tipperary. It is noticed that as a rule the first persons attacked are children, thence it spreads to adults, and a medical authority considers it much more difficult for adults to get over an attack than for children. When one is dealing with influenza there is only one way of dealing with it; go straight to bed and remain there until the attack has spent its force. But the best way to ward off an attack is to take plenty of exercise and fresh air and to avoid crowded places. One child, if affected, can communicate influenza to a hundred persons in a very short time. As to the cause of the present epidemic little is known. It is suggested that soldiers coming home on leave may have brought it from the front. But it first appeared in Spain, and one has not heard that it was prevalent in France, though a far-fetched explanation of the present German inactivity on the Western front is the suggestion that the enemy is suffering from influenza. Others blame the war for the outbreak, and many with more show of

reason, attribute it to the general food scarcity and the short commons to which all have to submit with the subsequent reduction of vitality, which weakens resistance to any epidemic.[10]

By the next day's newspaper reports, the sense of alarm was increasing, as the mysterious influenza plague had reached Dublin, where 200 cases had been reported. Dr Matthew J. Russell, assistant medical officer of health (MOH) for Dublin Corporation, stated that sixty children in one convent and forty employees in a factory had caught it. The symptoms, Russell noted, seemed mild enough – stiffness, feverishness, distaste for solid food, with vomiting. The manager of Glencree industrial school, Enniskerry, announced that children could not receive visitors for the present owing to the epidemic. Several fatal cases were reported from Belfast.[11]

As the 'new' influenza continued to spread, there was a continued sense that attempts were being made to manage news about the disease in order to limit panic. Russell's senior, Dublin's chief MOH, the hardworking eighty-eight-year-old Sir Charles Cameron, was trying to calm the situation when he told an *Irish Independent* reporter that the disease usually passed off in three or four days when the patient took to bed. 'Children were very subject to it. The disease is not serious enough to cause alarm.'[12] Cameron was an amiable and unassuming man who had worked assiduously since his first appointment in 1859 to improve the health of the people of Dublin, through improving sanitation and promoting better housing and disease controls.[13] His endeavours to improve the city's abysmal death rates in the nineteenth century had earned him universal respect, but still the rates exceeded other large cities of the Union, such as London, Glasgow and Liverpool. Throughout the epidemic, newspaper reporters sought his opinion on the current state of influenza affairs. He responded with sensible, calming advice, while working in the background to do everything he thought reasonable to limit the effects of the disease.

Towards the end of June, the authorities in Belfast believed they had actually managed to contain the epidemic, by disinfecting all buildings and by introducing other preventive measures. Large numbers of people were still ill in Lurgan, and in Derry many factory and shipyard workers had caught it.[14]

In early July, the newspapers were beginning to describe the spread of the disease in Dublin city and suburbs as 'alarming' and often

referred to it as plague. Likening it to plague had a significant reson-
ance, for in the fourteenth century, plague had caused an estimated
50 million deaths in Europe.[15] The disease was no longer considered
innocuous: two deaths had been recorded in the Dublin area; five or
six in Lurgan and thirty in Belfast. The authorities in Belfast were
reporting that the city had 100 deaths from complications of influenza. Some 100 motor-men and conductors on the Belfast trams were
reported to be off work. The previous weekend had seen numerous
flu deaths in Derry. The 'plague' was reported to be virulent in Cork,
with several people having fallen in the streets. In London, scores of
chemists had sold out of medicines. Ambulances there were said to be
very busy. About 70 per cent of all English employees were off work,
either through sickness or closure due to the illness.[16]

As Irish leader writers engaged themselves with trying to explain
the unusual presence of influenza in the summer months, they eagerly
read and quoted sources from other publications, keeping a watch on
its international progress, and trying to unpick the puzzles about this
disease and its diffusion. One cited a medical correspondent of the
Manchester Guardian as considering that

> the very mild February may have removed the barrage of cold which
> usually keeps the bacillus in Asia and allowed the epidemic to spread
> all over Europe. It was active on the Continent for some months,
> affecting the civilian population and soldiers alike, before it appeared
> in the United Kingdom, and it may be noticed that it gained a strong
> hold in England before it spread to Ireland.[17]

Others blamed it on dust from the unusually dry summer, or discussed
the likelihood of the Almighty having sent a great pestilence such
as influenza to put an end to the war. 'Parsons speak of it in their
sermons. It comes on many a wind of rumour. When we first heard
it from Spain that more than six millions of Spaniards were down
with influenza, we though this is surely the pestilence at last.' But a
physician interviewed by this leader writer in the *Midland Reporter*
poured cold water on such fanciful notions. 'No influenza of any type
we know could end this war, and this, obviously, is not at present of
the type which is dangerous.'[18]

From the middle of July, the threat from the first influenza epidemic of 1918 receded, and newspapers became preoccupied with
other issues. Common themes in the provincial newspapers were food

control orders, the milk and coal shortages, news of the Sinn Féin members imprisoned in Britain, and Sinn Féin's fundraising activities. There were still occasional reports of the first wave of the epidemic, particularly in more remote areas. Local notes for Edenderry in the *Midland Reporter and Westmeath Nationalist* on 8 August 1918 said that although the 'flue' (sic) had abated somewhat in the town, two further deaths had occurred. The paper's Longford notes reported that the epidemic was rife in the town, but no deaths had been reported.

The second wave – October 1918: Dublin and Wicklow

In early October, the Dublin-based *Evening Herald* noted that the epidemic of Spanish influenza in South Africa had severely disrupted mining, with gold production falling by 10 per cent. De Beers had suspended operations in the Dutoitspan mine. Government offices, harbours and businesses in Cape Town were severely disrupted by influenza.[19]

The *Evening Herald* reported on 7 October:

> The disease is really endemic. I am sorry to say that several doctors and nurses have been knocked up. The beastly thing spares none, but, of course the person in good average health and regular habits will stand a better chance of getting it light and of soon getting rid of it.

Schools in Dublin city and suburbs were severely affected by the epidemic. Several well-known singers had been infected. At Dublin port, several of the harbour staff and men working in other shore-side departments were ill, including the Harbour Master, Commander J.H. Webb, RNR.[20]

On 9 October, the *Herald* was filled with alarming reports of the influenza epidemic, under the headline 'Flu's death march'. There were said to be 180,000 new cases of Spanish influenza in the German Army, and 100,000 cases in Budapest alone. Outbreaks had happened in Lucerne, Lausanne, Geneva, Zurich, St. Gall and Boston. Again, Charles Cameron tried to maintain calm, telling a reporter that there was no cause for alarm in Dublin city, where there had only been four deaths from influenza in the previous fortnight. The death rate for that fortnight was one third less than the average of the corresponding fortnight for the previous ten years. The Howth outbreak was large; at a meeting that day of the recently amalgamated

North and South Dublin Boards of Guardians (BOGs) a second doctor was appointed to help out with patients there. The guardians empowered the relieving officer to appoint more practitioners for the Grand Canal Street Dispensary. The same paper reported that the dispute in the city's undertaking trade showed no change, and funerals were still being deferred. Trade disputes were a frequent topic in news pages. Increased costs of living, especially for food and fuel, were causing severe hardship to many workers, who sought to force pay increases by withholding their services. Concurrent trade disputes were taking place in the print industry, the Chapelizod distillery, among the cross-channel dockers at the port of Dublin and the engineering department workers of the Dublin port and docks board. The next day, Sir Charles Cameron admitted that epidemic influenza had appeared in several districts in the city, and advised that children should not be sent to school for the present.[21]

A German submarine torpedoed the mail steamer *Leinster* off the east coast as it made its way from Dun Laoghaire to Holyhead in Wales on 10 October 1918.[22] Influenza dropped in priority as newspapers dealt with the story of the *Leinster*. More than 500 of the 687 people on board died, including many members of the aristocracy and postal workers. National and provincial papers devoted hundreds of column inches to this atrocity over the following days, and carried harrowing stories of lives lost and saved, bodies recovered, funerals, memorial services, obituaries and relief funds.

The newspapers were still reacting to this impact of war on the doorstep when the *Irish Independent* reported that influenza was rife in the city and other places. Fourteen deaths from influenza in the city had been recorded at the offices of the Public Health Committee the same week, although the reporter pointed out that it was difficult to quantify the real number of deaths from influenza, as it was not a notifiable disease. Doctors were obliged to notify the Local Government Board (LGB) officers about deaths caused by certain infectious diseases, including cholera, typhoid, measles and smallpox. A dispensary doctor told an *Irish Independent* reporter that almost three quarters of the deaths of people up to the age of thirty were either directly attributable to influenza, or to diseases resulting from it. 'For the previous ten days the number of deaths from pneumonia within the city has been unprecedented. Pneumonia follows with startling rapidity the moment the necessary precautions were

relaxed.' A doctor who had been working day and night for the previous fortnight in the North Dock district expressed the view that the
death rate in the poorer quarters from influenza was largely a result
of malnutrition.[23]

This wave was already causing much more disruption than the
attack in summer. Some city schools were already closed, and those
that remained open were severely affected by absent staff and pupils.
Bray and Kingstown (now Dun Laoghaire) to the south of Dublin,
and Howth, Grange and Baldoyle on the north side were all badly
affected. MOHs in Howth had also reported between 400 and 500
cases in the last couple of weeks, with whole families being affected
by the disease, and there had been many deaths.[24]

At a meeting of the Joint Dublin BOG on 16 October 1918,
Dr Burke of Ringsend dispensary district requested medical assistance
to deal with the influenza cases. Approving his request, the chairman
said that the LGB inspector Dr Brown had recommended that
assistant medical officers be temporarily appointed during the epidemic wherever required. Dr Conroy of Howth Dispensary District
reported that there were still 400 cases in Howth and Baldoyle, and
asked for three nurses and another doctor to help him with the poor
who were suffering from influenza.[25]

Many of the staff at shipping businesses in the port were ill. One
docker told the *Herald*, 'I'm going home or to "the hospital" – I don't
know which to call it – as there are four of my family in bed with
the flu.' Sir Charles Cameron told the *Herald* that he had received a
letter from a city schoolteacher advocating the closing of the schools.
'Teachers', he wrote, 'are daily risking their lives in a vitiated atmos-
phere, but still managers are adamant. We are of the opinion that the
Commissioners should order the general closing down of the schools
until the end of the month.'[26]

The *Irish Times* did not record the second wave of influenza in
the greater Dublin region until the following day. Dr H.J. Rafferty,
the MOH for Bray number one district, reported to the Rathdown
Board of Guardians about a fresh epidemic of influenza in Bray,
involving about 600 cases in the previous days. In the midst of all
the coverage of the attack on the Leinster, the report only merited
three small paragraphs.[27] Rafferty's report was given rather more
coverage by the *Wicklow People* than the *Irish Times*. He warned the
board that 'ordinary methods' of treatment were quite inadequate to

deal with this influenza when fully developed. It was imperative to use preventive measures, especially a vaccine, and he urged the government to set scientific investigators working on one at once. 'The ravages are now greater than on the first occasion, and one can only view with horror the consequences of the present epidemic if it continues with its course unchecked', he stressed. The relieving officer for Bray, Patrick Dempsey, told the guardians that the previous Saturday, Rafferty visited seventy-four houses, in all 300 cases of influenza, with six or eight people in each house requiring attention. A rough calculation shows us that if Rafferty worked eighteen hours that day, he would have averaged sixteen patients and four households an hour, a phenomenal work rate, but one that is supported by other accounts as not being all that unusual during the pandemic. Rafferty asked the relieving officer to get extra medical help. Two days later, Dempsey had had to appoint two more doctors as the situation had worsened, and they had dealt with perhaps 600 cases since Saturday.[28] The Rathdown guardians sent a wire to the LGB: 'Terrible influenza epidemic in whole Rathdown district; 600 alone in Bray affected; union full; several deaths; immediate action of LGB requested.'[29] The LGB responded – by post – suggesting that the sanitary authorities of Rathdown Numbers 1 and 2 Rural Councils might get volunteers to visit houses in their areas where there were patients. There was a shortage of nurses anyhow, but because of the epidemic it would be impracticable to obtain a large number of trained nurses to assist the medical officers. In any case if the medical officer could not cope it was up to the relieving officer to get help for him. Dempsey made the rather pointed reply that he had already appointed six doctors in addition to Rafferty, spurred on by a threat from Drs Rowntree and Hanson on 18 October to be relieved of their duties if other doctors were not appointed, as they would not hold themselves responsible for so many cases.[30]

Rafferty's report to the Rathdown Board of Guardians and the response of the LGB raised issues that were to become common themes in reports about influenza from other BOGs around the country: manpower and vaccines, appeals to the Government authorities to take action, and the LGB's apparent belief that influenza was a local issue where it occurred and was better dealt with by local authorities rather than by a central body. Boards of guardians and medical officers in many parts of the country were soon appealing for extra doctors to treat all the ill. They also repeatedly urged the Government to investigate the disease and search for an effective vaccine.[31] Professor Culverwell of Trinity College, Dublin wrote to several newspapers extolling the virtues of a vaccine he had developed, and offering to send supplies to 'any medical man interested.' He suggested that 'in the meantime, all bacteriological laboratories ought to be employed making stocks of vaccine.'[32] The national newspapers did not record any response from the LGB to Culverwell's proposals.

In the third week in October, the *Evening Herald* reported that the city ambulances were busily removing pneumonia cases to hospital, and in some instances both a father and a mother were taken to hospital at the same time. Often every member of the family was affected. Hospitals were crowded with cases, but were handicapped by the fact that in many instances their staff were depleted by the epidemic. The Sisters of Charity transformed the schools at Ravenswell, Little Bray, into a hospital for children suffering from the epidemic. Appeals were made in several places for funds to help the sick poor. Several school teachers had died from pneumonia contracted at work. Some of the schools were closed; in those schools that were still open, many pupils were missing. The staff of many business houses were also ill. In the Dublin Metropolitan Police (DMP), 114 men were under medical care, mostly with influenza, and three had died. The E Division had twenty-seven members who were ill, as against ten to twenty from other divisions.[33]

In the leading article on 21 October, the *Herald* mentions that public health authorities in the United States had systematically organised a campaign for dealing with the scourge, closing theatres, picture-houses and schools, and giving the public a warning of the dangers of infection posed by large gatherings. They also mobilised 4,000 graduate and attendant nurses to meet the needs of the sufferers, and had arranged to move nursing units from city to city, where they were most urgently required. The American authorities were also endeavouring to find a cure. The *Herald* writer scolded the authorities in Ireland for not behaving in a similarly responsible way:

> Sir Charles Cameron himself admits it is the most dangerous epidemic of the kind that has every visited the city. We have no desire whatever to create alarm, but facts should be faced and the most effective measures

concerted to combat the scourge in our midst. We notice this morning that the Commissioners of National Education have tardily decided to authorise Dublin managers to close their schools for a fortnight. That is an obvious precaution, and we hope that where it has not yet been taken up it will now be put into operation without further delay. We are ... justified in this connection in asking the question: Whether our Public Health Authorities are doing everything possible to combat this malignant and widespread disease? ... The problem which at this moment affects the health authorities is a very grave one, and no effort or expense should be spared in the endeavour to cope with it. A policy of drift or an attitude of *laissez faire* in such an emergency cannot be tolerated, and the battle against disease must be organised on systematic and thorough lines. The urgency of the matter must be apparent to everyone.

In Dublin, Sir Charles Cameron closed the schools as the epidemic progressed. Criticised by some for taking this measure, he was also reprimanded by others for not going further and also closing theatres, picture houses and music halls. 'I only did what every health officer does under similar conditions', he wrote to the editor of the *Irish Independent*.[34] 'Last week there were 66 deaths due to influenza, and 22 victims were children. In the townships the mortality appears to be greater.' The newspapers were full of conjecture and debate about what measures should be taken, and sometimes of who to blame. Between the first and the twenty-first of October, 490 people were buried in Glasnevin Cemetery, compared with 243 in the corresponding period in 1917. This represented a daily average of twenty-three burials since the epidemic re-emerged in Dublin, as against normal interments averaging twelve a day. Towards the end of this three-week period, as many as forty bodies were buried in the cemetery in a day. The epidemic was reaching its peak in the city. The following week, 343 were buried in Glasnevin, almost as many as had died on the *Leinster*.[35]

Cameron, his assistant (Dr Russell), and Mr P.T. Daly (the chairman of the Public Health Committee) visited Dublin hospitals on 23 October to assess the accommodation available for influenza patients. They found that many of the beds were occupied by soldiers – the army had an arrangement with several hospitals to provide beds for soldiers – and decided to approach the military authorities to ask them to provide other accommodation for military patients. The military authorities agreed not to send soldiers to civilian hospitals with effect from 24 October. Asked about the vaccine treatment of the flu, Cameron said that so far as Dublin experience went the use of vaccine had had favourable results, but he did not think that any positive opinion could be formed yet on the subject.[36]

One of the constant themes in the newspapers was that despite the shortage of doctors, four doctors were either interned or 'on the run'; politicians and journalists called for them to be allowed to work during the crisis. Alderman Thomas Kelly told a Dublin Corporation meeting that three doctors had been interned, at a time when there was a severe shortage of doctors to treat the ill. He was referring to 'German' plot internees Dr Hayes, MOH with South Dublin Union, and Dr Cusack and Dr McNabb. He also appealed for Dr Kathleen Lynn, known for her work with the sick poor, to be allowed to come off 'the run'. His sentiments were to be echoed at many other local authority and board of guardian meetings in the following days. Father Murray, chaplain of the Mater Hospital, fell ill while ministering to the hospital's influenza patients, and died from pneumonia. Alderman J.J. Kelly, JP, adjourned for a month the sitting of the Children's (Street Trading) Court, deferring over 100 cases. Dublin Corporation's Cleansing Committee began disinfecting the streets and gullies on 26 October.[37]

Stories of people becoming disoriented and meeting with mishap while suffering from influenza were commonplace, in newspapers and in private memories. They seemed to happen as ill people struggled to continue with daily life. Some stumbled under trams or carriages, or collapsed in the street. The *Evening Herald* documented the sad story of a Donnybrook man who walked into the shallow pond at Herbert Park and drowned while suffering from a high fever with influenza, on his way to get medicine for himself and his ill wife.[38]

Deep into the second wave, the doubts about whether this unusual flu actually was flu continued to emerge in the press. A *Herald* reporter wrote: 'Some doubt is felt, even by doctors, that the epidemic raging is solely influenza. There is no question but that we have veritable influenza amongst us … but the violence of the attack and the high mortality in many households gives colour to the suggestion that combined with influenza is a deadly malady not yet identified.'[39]

Catholic Church authorities considered the outbreak so severe that the Archbishop of Dublin, William Walsh, wrote to his people appealing to them not to weaken themselves by observing fast or abstinence for the Vigil of the Feast of All Saints on 31 October.

He issued instructions to reduce the number of prayers at funeral masses, and even ordered that the corpse should not be brought into the church if the risk of infection was considered too great.[40]

As the flu reached its zenith in Dublin in the last week of October and beginning of November, there was an evident anxiety about its effects on the police forces. In response to a parliamentary question by Mr Nugent, the chief commissioner of the DMP, T.E. Johnston provided the information (for the Chief Secretary's reply) that so far eight members of the force had died from the epidemic. All serious cases were sent to hospital. In each barrack, rooms had been set apart for the use of those afflicted. The force's three medical officers had been in constant attendance on the sick men. All men who were willing to be inoculated with the vaccine had received it. All barracks were being disinfected daily; the men received full pay during their illness, as well as free medical attendance and medicine.[41] By 2 November, the *Irish Times* reported that 210 members of the DMP were in hospital, and that eight members had died in the previous three weeks.

The normally restrained *Irish Times* described, in the issue of 31 October 1918, the dramaturgy of the influenza, as hearse after hearse passed through the streets of the city to the cemeteries:

> Yesterday, from early morning till well after midday, cortege after cortege reached Glasnevin Cemetery, sometimes as many as three corpse-laden hearses being seen proceeding up Sackville Street at the same time. Close on forty orders for interment were issued at the Cemeteries' Office yesterday, and, inclusive of the remains brought for burial on the previous day, which had been temporarily placed in the vaults overnight, there were close on one hundred bodies for sepulchre. At Mount Jerome there were eight interments – a number much in excess of the daily average.[42]

By 2 November, epidemic conditions became so severe the *Irish Times* abandoned its reserved coverage. Under atypically large headlines of INFLUENZA EPIDEMIC IN IRELAND – HEAVY DEATH TOLL; EFFORTS TO COMBAT THE DISEASE, it documented the difficulties with trade, as business houses and factories found it difficult to stay open because so many of their staff were ill. Doctors, nurses and chemists were in heavy demand, and working all hours, and hospital accommodation everywhere was severely taxed. Official figures showed that hundreds of people had died in Dublin during the month, with 231 dying during the week ending 25 October. There was a practically unbroken succession of funeral processions on their way to Glasnevin Cemetery. On several days, the Cemeteries' Committee employees could not do all the interments, and had to resort to storing bodies overnight in the vault; it was reported that the cemeteries had not been so busy since the cholera outbreak of the 1830s. The cemeteries' staff had done 232 burials in separate graves, and eighty-two in the area reserved for burying paupers. Mount Jerome had buried fifty-five for the week ended 29 October, against eleven in the corresponding week in 1917. Of these deaths, thirty-four were certified to pneumonia or influenza. Even though cinema houses and places of entertainment were being disinfected, there had been a marked drop in attendances. Business people in the city complained of a trade paralysis. One leading grocer remarked that the great bulk of his customers were sending in written orders by messenger rather than coming to collect them themselves. In turn, he said, this placed a burden on the regular delivery service, as the orders were coming in hundreds rather than in the regular dozens. Businesses were being liberally sprinkled with antiseptic fluids. Druggists reported having had such big orders that stocks ran out.

On 10 December 1918, the *Irish Independent* and the *Evening Herald* paper covered the story of the death of 'German' plot internee Richard Coleman's death, just before the pivotal general election. In subsequent days the newspapers documented the draping of Sinn Féin election flags in Balbriggan, Swords and Dublin city with black crêpe to mourn Richard Coleman, and described the preparations for his elaborate funeral procession through the city centre to Glasnevin Cemetery.[43]

As the second wave of the epidemic waned during November, the newspapers again turned their attention to other issues, including coverage of the end of the war and the Paris Peace Conference, and the general election. Thirty-six of the seventy-three Sinn Féin members of parliament and other party activists were still interned in Britain, and it was difficult to get news about them. In late January 1919, George Lyons was sent home to Dublin because of ill health. He gave an interview to the *Irish Independent* about conditions in the prison. The internees' only opportunity for exercise was in a yard measuring ten feet by sixty-three, which they considered totally inadequate for twenty men. Most of the young men who had been used to an athletic life had become limp and useless; the confinement and the restless state of mind of the men owing to repeated rumours of release had also reduced their mental activity. The influenza epidemic was virulent. The prison officers themselves were first infected, and ultimately the governor. The prison doctor was away at the front and the doctor responsible could only pay casual visits, having over 200 cases to attend to in the town. Mellowes caught it on 27 November, followed by J.J. Clancy on the twenty-eighth, and K. Moone and Joseph McGrath on the twenty-ninth. Richard Coleman and Willie Brennan Whitmore became ill on 30 November. On 1 December a resident doctor arrived. A new prison hospital was opened the next day, and the invalids were removed there. On 6 December, a nurse came to assist the medical officer for an hour a day. 'Up to this time', Lyons said, 'the nursing was being done by ourselves, and we were naturally contracting the disease, delicate men stopping up at night to attend to their comrades.' Coleman died on 9 December; his emotional comrades carried his corpse late at night, in a downpour of rain, over two prison yards to their wing of the prison. Lyons added that the condition of two other prisoners, Whitmore and Donovan, was still causing anxiety.[44]

The reportage of the second wave of the influenza epidemic by the Leinster regional newspapers follows a broadly similar pattern; by then, journalists and the public alike were familiar with the disease. It is reported that the flu has arrived, that there is scarcely a family unaffected in the town. The schools, cinemas and other public buildings are closed, for some weeks, the court sittings adjourned. The Poor Law BOGs' meetings invariably have a report from the master of the workhouse or the fever hospital stating that the premises are full and that they are having trouble finding staff; the relieving officer too reports that he is having difficulty in finding doctors to replace those who are ill, and that he has to offer increasingly larger fees to persuade doctors to work for him. In some areas, a local official or group shows initiative and takes it on themselves to take measures to prevent the spread or provide community care for the ill, with some comment about the absence of any great help from the central government. There is a list of the numbers who are ill, and usually a couple of columns of obituaries to the week's influenza victims. These columns usually include athletes of some kind, shopkeepers and their assistants, priests and doctors. The athletes are always included with comments about how unlikely it was that young, fit people should die. The other categories may have been included simply because they were well known locally through their work, or perhaps, because by virtue of that work, they were more likely to come into contact with the virus.

The second wave: Kildare

Doctors, who were always in the frontline dealing with the influenza crisis, frequently caught the flu; under pressure because of a shortage of physicians and nurses, many tried to continue working beyond the point at which it was wise to do so. During the week ending Saturday, 19 October 1918, several cases had to be adjourned at Naas Quarter Sessions, owing to the absence of doctors whose evidence was considered necessary. All three Naas doctors – Coady, Murphy and Browne, were confined to bed during the past week, as a result of contraction of the disease during their professional ministrations.[45] Others, through their work with the public, were also effectively at the frontline: policemen, nurses, priests, shopkeepers and their assistants were frequently victims. The columns of obituaries in the provincial newspapers pay testimony to these lost lives. They also show clusters of deaths in occupations: in Naas there was a particularly bad out-break of flu among the staff of the *Leinster Leader*, with the foreman printer, W.R. Blackford, and a bookbinder, E. Slater, dying.

Kildare, with its rail and canal links and strong socio-economic ties to the metropolitan area, was affected almost simultaneously with Dublin and Wicklow. The county had the worst death toll per head from influenza in 1918. The *Irish Independent* reported that the district of Naas, Co. Kildare, had a remarkably high incidence of influenza, and several young people died between 8 October and 18 October. By the week ending 26 October, the *Kildare Observer* was reporting that scarcely a family in Naas that has not been afflicted:

> In too many cases, death has claimed his victims. Pneumonia supervenes in quite a number of cases, possibly through the reluctance of the victim to take warning in time. Many of the doctors have fallen victim to the flu and the demands on the services of those who remain leave little or no time for the ordinary night's rest. Inconvenience has been added in business places and in the domestic circle by the absence of gas for lighting, cooking or power purposes. The whole of

the Naas Gas Co.'s staff has been put out o'action by the flu, with the result that you may or may not have gas to cook your meals, to drive your machinery, or to light your home or office. It certainly does seem a little strange that the Gas Co, realising the seriousness of the position in a town where three-fourths of its inhabitants are dependent on gas for lighting and where business has to be suspended in the absence of gas should not have made provision for procuring a temporary staff within the last few days.[46]

Illness among Naas Gas Company's staff put serious pressure on the town. Businesses were only receiving a sporadic supply of gas to fuel their machinery; the *Kildare Observer* had particular cause to complain: it had to run with blank pages in one issue because it only had four hours' supply of gas during the week.

The gas supply was not the only local issue that the flu exacerbated, as the *Kildare Observer*'s writers eagerly pointed out. The urban district council's regulations on water meant that the water supply to the town was cut off at night, which interfered with the treatment of the disease. Part of the treatment for pneumonia was regular poulticing, which required hot water, and Naas residents could not obtain water at night.[47] The *Kildare Observer* also used the epidemic to raise the issue of the pail system of sewage disposal still operating in parts of the town.

Naas is not the only town in Ireland seriously affected by the dreadful malady, but we venture to suggest that in few towns have the number of deaths been so great as in this town. If we add to the fact that a prehistoric system of domestic scavenging – the pail system – is still permitted to continue in many parts of the town, the undesirable proximity to the middle of the town of a refuse depot that is at no time maintained in a sanitary condition, we have a state of things of which Naas has no reason to be proud.[48]

The epidemic had allowed the focus to fall on the pail system, which the journalist considered was little short of a scandal when it was possible to connect all houses to a flush system.[49] Criticism in the local press was a powerful catalyst for the urban district council – at its next meeting it approved the provision of limewash to disinfect houses and disinfectant for the rubbish dump.

The Naas branch of the Women's National Health Association (WNHA) set up a communal kitchen to provide free soups and stews to the ill poor and their relatives. The kitchen opened each day at the town hall from 11am to 1pm, and the WNHA appealed for contributions of food and money to support it.[50] The St Vincent de Paul Society was also helped out[51] Another communal kitchen was set up in Athy by local ladies at the request of Athy Urban District Council, feeding the afflicted with hot soup, gruel and milk at the local technical school, which was closed because of the epidemic. At the peak of its operations this communal kitchen fed sixty-one men, 336 women and 445 children, the Athy Board of Guardians reported. The chairman of the board, Thomas Plewman, said that the fifty deaths in the town in the previous three weeks might have been 150 but for the voluntary help given by the ladies of the town.[52]

As the influenza crisis in Kildare continued, the *Kildare Observer* complained about the Government's 'attitude of almost supineness towards a malady which has been the cause of a tremendous death toll. This government inertia ... should not be allowed to go on without at least a serious effort being made in the battle with the disease'.[53] Given the polarised state of political affairs at the time of the epidemic, and given also that reporting, including that of the deaths of influenza victims, was coloured by politics, it is interesting to note that the pro-establishment *Observer* voiced some of the harshest criticisms of the Government's strategy, or rather its perceived lack of strategy, to deal with the disease. The *Observer's* peculiar readership catchment area would have included areas in north Kildare, where several members of the Ascendancy with extensive and close political connections to the Government lived, among them the Bartons at Straffan House and the Earl of Mayo at Palmerstown House, near Naas; the Curragh army base would also have been in its catchment area. Co. Kildare had the highest per capita death rate in the country in 1918. The high rate of illness, combined with the crippling of Naas' industry and commerce by the lack of power, seemed to steer the *Observer* and its nationalist rival, the *Leinster Leader*, more towards campaigning journalism than any other newspaper within Leinster. They not only criticised the political leadership but also called for targeted voluntary action to replace the services the Government had, they considered, failed to provide, and debated the merits and flaws of methods of treatment and vaccination.

The *Observer* engaged in thorough reportage of the vaccination issues. It reported that many people had said they would like to be vaccinated but were put off by the cost, which was rumoured to be 30s or £2 a head. The columnist had interviewed an unnamed doctor from

Trinity College who said that the £2 bottle actually covered thirty people. He also was told that many people were not actually suffering from the flu but from fear.[54]

By mid-November, the peak of the epidemic had passed in County Kildare. Dr Morrissey reported to the Naas Board of Guardians that when he had been called to Naas on 13 October there were between 300 and 400 cases of flu in the town; a week later there were 1,000 cases. By 26 October there were 1,420 cases in Naas and immediate districts. Considering the severity of the disease, he did not consider the death toll to be too high; out of a population of 4,000, about one in one hundred died, he believed.[55]

The second wave: Louth

The second wave arrived in Dundalk a week later than Naas, Bray and Dublin. By 23 October 1918 there were nearly 1,100 cases of influenza reported, nearly one in ten of the population. Again, as elsewhere, the doctors were reported to have been worked off their feet. Two of them, Dr Flood and Dr O'Hagan, became ill early in the week, and the other doctors were attending hundreds of cases daily. The number of deaths was reported in the *Dundalk Democrat and People's Journal* to be alarming. To prevent the spread of the disease, the urban council on the advice of the doctors ordered the closing of the schools, picture houses, and so on, for three weeks from 23 October. Several cases listed for hearing at Dundalk Petty Sessions were adjourned owing to the parties being laid up with influenza.[56]

As in Kildare, Wicklow and Dublin, the deaths included the young and fit, not normally badly affected by influenza. One of the victims was cycling ace and Louth county footballer Joe Ross, who left a wife and five young children. According to the *Dundalk Democrat and People's Journal*: 'It would be harder to find a finer specimen of physical fitness than poor Joe Ross, the cycling crack, who succumbed after a very hard fight on Wednesday. In three or four cases the mothers of young families were taken – the case of the soldier's wife [Mrs Lucy Lawrence] who was found dead in the bed with her weeping infants beside her is peculiarly sad.' The paper also commented on the youthful deaths of veterinary surgeon Patrick McDonnell and his wife Mary. 'Both Mr and Mrs. McDonnell were young strong healthy people and their deaths show how virulent is the disease which is now ravaging this community as well as others in Ireland.' They left a young family.[57]

The *Democrat* also reported Professor Culverwell's claim to have developed an effective vaccine for influenza: 'Professor Culverwell offers to take steps to enable any medical man communicating with him to obtain a supply of the vaccine, and suggests that all the bacteriological laboratories ought to be employed in making stocks of vaccine. What are the public health authorities at the Custom House doing about this?'[58]

The *SS Dundalk* was sunk by a German submarine on a voyage from Liverpool to Dundalk. Twenty-one Irish seamen and crew were killed or missing. Survivors took to boats in mid-channel, some of them ended up in Holyhead and in Douglas. Three of the missing men were on their first tour of duty on the *Dundalk*, as some of regular crew were off sick. During the week two members of the standing crew of the vessel had died from pneumonia following influenza, Patrick R(e)ddy and Patrick Hanratty. When the *Dundalk* was torpedoed Hanratty's dead body was being taken across for burial in his native town.[59] Patrick Kearney of Dowdallshill, temporary charge cattleman on the *Dundalk*, described his own struggle to survive. He was woken during the night by a tremendous noise, finding the ship split in two and sinking by the head. He and his companions in the deck cabin rushed to the lifeboats. They rescued two gunners who were clinging on to some floating wreckage. 'One of them had been laid up with the influenza and was very sick. He was clad only in a singlet and drawers, suffered horrible from the cold in the water, and was helpless when taken into the boat.' They spent seventeen hours in the open boat, two of them baling out the boat which had been damaged by the explosion. Everyone else rowed while the sick gunner directed them to the Welsh coast by compass.[60]

By 2 November, the number of influenza cases in Dundalk had risen to 2,000. The schools in the town remained closed, and the book lending department of the Free Library was closed for a fortnight. More than half the staff of the Post Office were off ill. The *Democrat* urged the charitable ladies of the town to set up a food depot to provide beef tea and other food to families where the mother was laid up. Thirty people were believed to have died so far, mostly previously healthy young people. They included three adult daughters of Patrick Eaton, a compositor who worked for the *Democrat*. The following week, the paper reported that the epidemic was rapidly declining in Dundalk, with the number ill down to between three and four hundred, compared to over 2,000 the previous week. Four of the town's doctors, Dr O'Hagan, Dr O'Connell, Dr Flood and Dr Clarke, had influenza.

The following week, the *Democrat* reported that a communal kitchen had been set up in the technical schools. Volunteers cooked soup, beef tea and Irish stew and barley water, and people came to collect them for sick friends, neighbours and families whose mother was 'down and out'. Messages came from doctors and others about people who needed the food, and more volunteers distributed it. A small fee was charged to cover the cost of the food. Some local farmers sent potatoes. As well as running a communal kitchen, the group set up a nursing committee to train girls to nurse their families or neighbours.[61]

Doctors told the *Democrat* that they were trying to control influenza hysteria, a danger in itself. One doctor advised that there was nothing very serious in the disease if precautionary measures were taken, and if people took to their bed as soon as they got symptoms. 'In some of the country districts people are becoming greatly alarmed at the spread of the disease ... there is a danger that the people may become panic stricken by even unexaggerated accounts of the ravages of the epidemic and thus help on the disease.'[62]

On 14 November, James Toal, Bachelor's Walk, Dundalk, one of the Sinn Féin leaders in the district, died from pneumonia. Mr Toal had been imprisoned earlier in the year on the charge of unlawful assembly. Over 6,000 people accompanied his remains for burial to St Patrick's cemetery in Dundalk.[63]

The second wave: Kilkenny

The *Kilkenny People* offered the following advice to its readers in mid-October 1918:

> Regular meals to keep the body in peak condition, and if you get home wet or late take a hot glass of lemonade immediately. Inhale eucalyptus from a piece of cotton wool several times a day. Go to bed immediately if you get the flu. It is no exaggeration to say that half the people who die directly or indirectly from influenza owe their fate to the imprudence of fighting the disease.[64]

Influenza had become the newspaper's main story by the following week. The following leading article appeared under the banner headline 'THE FLU IN KILKENNY – MANY SUFFERERS':

> The mysterious epidemic is once more rampant around the city ... it has spread to an alarming extent within the past week, and caused numerous deaths wherever it has reached. The number of victims in Kilkenny, especially among the young people, is very high, and there is scarcely a family in the city that has escaped its ravages. In some streets there were but one or two members of the family left untouched, and in many cases the attack has developed into pneumonia. There are many instances of people suddenly collapsing in the streets on their way to or from work. The county and workhouse infirmaries are crowded with people suffering from the disease. Early in the week the Christian Brothers' schools, James's Street, were compelled to close, as the majority of the brothers and pupils were confined to bed with influenza, and the concerts to be held last night and tonight in aid of the schools had to be postponed for the same reason. Several of the Brothers of St Patrick's schools are also suffering. On Wednesday all the schools of the city were closed on the recommendation of the mayor and the corporation, who were advised by the medical officers of health for the city that it would help lessen the danger of infection. Fortunately there have been few deaths in the city up to the present attributable to the disease, but we understand that there are a large number of people in a very dangerous condition.[65]

By 2 November, the newspaper was describing the extent of the 'so-called influenza epidemic's ravages (as) abnormal, and the high death rate attributed to it as alarming'. The Kilkenny Union BOG agreed to double the outdoor relief provision from 1 November to 1 January for the city and for country districts where necessary, at the request of the city's mayor, John Slater, to alleviate hardship caused by the awful outbreak of influenza. The mayor said that the disease was affecting rich and poor alike. The meeting also mentioned the shortage of provisions like milk and coal as another problem for impoverished influenza sufferers. It was also agreed to appoint another doctor to help the two medical officers of health. An urban district council meeting mentioned the milk shortage in the context of the influenza outbreak. The council had posted notices advising people to keep away from crowded places. Streets were sprayed with the disinfectant carbolicine. The meeting was told that there were several cases in the town where entire families were stricken with no one to take care of them, and that there was also a problem appointing nurses, the job of the Union's relieving officer, as he had the flu.[66]

The epidemic, according to the newspaper, first made its appearance in Kilkenny ten days previously, and had initially confined itself to the younger people. The *Kilkenny People* went into a lot of detail about the dead: Philip Hogan from St John's Cottage, Kilkenny died at a private hospital in Dublin from pneumonia following an attack of influenza. Mr Hogan was a rate collector and an auctioneer with a large business. He left a wife and two young children. Other deaths mentioned were of Philip Clohosey, the thirteen-year-old son of Alderman Clohosey, John Street and Parliament St, Kilkenny, Thomas King of Butt's Green, a young man who ran a bakery, grocery and general business with his sister, and George Cullen, the chief warder at Kilkenny Prison. William Timmins, Nore Terrace, Dublin Road, Kilkenny, a commercial traveller in Carlow and Queen's County for Messrs O'Hanrahan and Company, Irishtown, also died. Chrissie Brophy, an assistant in the Brennan and O'Brien's drapery, High Street was another victim. A mechanic at Messrs Statham and Co. Kilkenny, Patrick Hehir, and a young man named Kennedy who worked as an assistant in E.J. Delahunty's Ironmongery and Engineering works, High Street, Miss Doheny, an assistant in O'Keefe's confectionary shop, High Street, and Mr M. Carrigan, Clara, an assistant at D.J. Stapleton's Medical Hall, High Street, were other victims. This particular list – of shop assistants, auctioneers, commercial travellers, prison warders – suggests that jobs which brought people into close contact with the public made people more vulnerable to catching the disease.[67]

The *Kilkenny People* of 9 November 1918 reported many more deaths in Kilkenny city. Business premises remained closed, hospitals crowded, clergy and doctors working day and night. Cinemas, schools and theatres also closed. At the Carnegie Libraries, books returned since the epidemic were being kept separate, and no more books were being issued. Mr O'Grady of the Urban District Council (UDC) said that he would ask the priests to get the churches sprayed with carbolicene before Sunday masses. The libraries had also been disinfected.[68]

That week's influenza victims included a shop assistant at Tynan's grocery, Mr James Hoyne, dentist Mr Williamson of John Street, and the wife of Mr M. Hickey, a shop assistant at Lipton's on High Street, alderman Thomas Cantwell, JP, who had a hardware and iron business on King Street, and James Pollard, the twenty-three-year-old owner of a grocer, hardware and timber merchant's business in Callan. A mother and her son, from Mullinavat, having been accused of the murder of the son's wife, were both reported to have the disease, as were both solicitors involved on the case. The Committee of the Grocers' Assistants' Section of the Irish Transport and General Workers' Union (Kilkenny) sent their sympathies to the families of five members of the section, Denis Brennan, James Hoyne, Robert Butler, William Kennedy and William Timmins, who had succumbed to the epidemic.

On 9 November, the newspaper carried a notice for chemists' shops showing the extended opening hours; from Monday 14 October 1918, they would close on weekdays at 8 pm, on Saturday at 10 pm; Sunday opening hours were 1 to 2 pm and 6 to 7 pm.

In mid-November, the MOHs in Kilkenny city told the local reporters that the epidemic had begun to abate; the cinema was to reopen, and the management said that the premises would be disinfected daily. Deaths were still frequent: the recent victims included Revd Fr Chrysostom Sutton, aged forty-one, OSFC at the Franciscan Friary, Kilkenny, the manageress of Power's Temperance Hotel, Miss Bridget Egan and butcher Mr Patrick Hickey of High Street.[69]

Three quarters of the staff of Kilkenny district asylum were reported to have been ill with influenza during November; one attendant died. Thomastown continued to be free of influenza at the end of the month, but in Graiguenamanagh, the disease was so prevalent that entire Royal Irish Constabulary police force in the town were sufferers and the barrack was closed until three members of the Thomastown force arrived.[70]

The second wave in Wexford

By the time the second wave reached Wexford county, Belfast, Dublin and Kildare had already experienced heavy losses from the disease, as the *People* and the *Enniscorthy Guardian* reported apprehensively.[71]

Gorey and New Ross were the first Wexford towns to be affected, in the third week of October. Within days, the newspapers were reporting that there was scarcely a house in Gorey without some member who was ill. The workhouse infirmary was almost full; some of the patients were the nursing staff and five members of the Royal Irish Constabulary (RIC) from the town.[72] The flu was still raging in Gorey a week later. The medical officer reported to the Gorey Board of Guardians that well over 200 people were affected; the workhouse hospital was full, and in some cases whole families were suffering, with no one in the household that was well enough to care for them.[73]

In New Ross, the picture seemed bleaker still. By 2 November, some 300 cases had been treated in the infirmary and forty in the Haughton hospital, and there had been 950 cases in all. Several of the nursing sisters, six policemen and Dr O'Regan had been ill as well, and a doctor had to be brought in from Dublin until Dr O'Regan resumed duty. As in other districts, local doctors were praised by journalists for their heroic work, having gone without sleep to tend to their patients. Some shops and all schools in the town and some rural districts were closed. Thirty-eight people had already died from the disease in the town, the infirmary and in Rosbercon. It was reported that in a few cases the faces of the victims became discoloured shortly after their death.[74]

Several deaths had been reported from influenza in Wexford town also by the beginning of November, and the disease was reported to be spreading there rapidly. All the schools in the town were closed and were being disinfected. The corporation was considering flushing the streets with disinfectant. Many of the ill were children, and several shop workers were 'down'. The MOH, Dr Pierse, reported to the Wexford Guardians that there were 200 cases in the town. A few days later, he told *The People* that he had no hesitation in affirming that there were about a thousand people under medical treatment, or one twelfth of the population. He strongly advised against attending the wakes of victims.[75] Wakes are an important part of the Irish funerary tradition. Before the body is removed to church, people come to pay their respects to the dead and their family in their home. Hospitality, usually in the form of sandwiches, cake, tea and sometimes alcohol, is offered. The body is usually uncoffined, laid out on a bed dressed in fine linen, surrounded by religious artefacts and often candles. Visitors spend some time in the room with the dead person, praying and talking quietly, and then move to another room to receive refreshments and tell of events in the dead person's life. Wakes can last one or more nights, and often relations and close friends of the dead will stay with the body overnight. Wakes can attract crowds in a small space, and therefore offer an opportunity for diseases like influenza to spread.

In Enniscorthy, townspeople were taking rigid precautions to prevent the disease from taking a grip in the town. All kinds of disinfectants were being used. 'Every second person one meets reeks of eucalyptus, while in the schools and buildings disinfectants are liberally used. Everything that medical science could suggest is being done with the view of minimising the effects of the disease', a *People* reporter wrote. The clergy in Enniscorthy cathedral had wisely decided to postpone the annual retreat for the local confraternities for fear of spreading germs.

Local businesses advertised their influenza-combating products in the papers. Readers of the *Enniscorthy Guardian* were urged to 'pour a little Cousins' lemonade into a saucepan and warm it, to provide the perfect drink for influenza sufferers'. A pharmacist in Gorey, James E. Cooke, claimed that his cod liver oil emulsion could protect against the influenza.

Enniscorthy's precautions may have had some effect, as it was the last major urban centre in the county to get cases of the flu, towards the end of the first week of November. An *Enniscorthy Guardian* journalist gave the following advice to the readers:

> No particular remedy has been decided on … the safest course is for the persons to go to bed immediately and take hot drinks, when the first symptoms appear and remain in bed until all traces are gone or until the doctor claims the patient may do so safely. As well as the ordinary influenza of a very severe type, some patients have been suddenly prostrated with illness, and when they succumbed their bodies become quickly discoloured. Many question whether this can be called influenza.[76]

This doubt about the diagnosis of influenza is a common theme in many of the newspapers. The Wexford papers were among the few who reported the cyanosis typical of the more extreme forms of Spanish influenza.

The People reported:

> Many persons have been confined to bed with the malady, which appears to be coming more severe. Delirium, feverishness, headache, stomach troubles and general pains have characterised it. Then in a few instances people have succumbed after a few hours' illness, and their bodies have become discoloured and have had to be coffined. Nothing has happened in this country so general and so severe for generations; there must be more than fifteen hundred cases down in Wexford a present.

By 16 November there were over 300 people who were ill in Enniscorthy town and district, and twelve people had died the previous week. The death rate was still reported to be light compared to that experienced in other districts. Dr Kelly, MOH, also advised against the holding of wakes, and that further suggested the bodies of people from the town and district who had died from the disease elsewhere should not be brought home for interment. All the town schools were closed, and many children were ill. The week's victims included Edward Ryan and Joseph O'Leary, who were both shop assistants. Five of the local police were on the sick list, and one doctor. Two priests had recovered; new sufferers included Canon O'Connor, who was the parish priest of Courtnacuddy, his curate, Revd Lennon, and Revd McCormack of Kiltealy.[77]

Coping strategies to deal with the influenza crisis were the main subject of discussion at a meeting of the Enniscorthy Board of Guardians in the second week of November. Dr Thomas Kelly had written to the board to explain he was overwhelmed by the work. It was decided to appoint an additional doctor, Dr John Pierse, son of the Wexford MOH, to assist him.[78]

Fear of contracting the disease did not prevent celebration of the ending of the war – the Germans had signed the armistice on Monday, 11 November. In Enniscorthy bonfires were lit in the Shannon, the Duffry and Fairfield districts, and crowds gathered to sing songs and cheer for the success of the Allies.

By the end of the second week of November, the epidemic was abating in Gorey, with only a few new cases during the week. But there had been several recent deaths. Two were young children belonging to Mr Peter Doran, a draper in Gorey, who also caught it himself.[79] Others who died during the week included the wife of Charles

O'Carroll, a chemist on the Main Street, and Mrs Thomas Byrne, a shopkeeper on Upper Main Street. By the end of the third week, only eighteen people in the Enniscorthy police district were reported to be newly 'down' with influenza. The county's champion handballer, Dan Farrell, died from pneumonia a few weeks after an apparent recovery. No fresh cases had been reported in Enniscorthy town during the week, but both doctors Murphy and Kelly were still extremely busy tending to the ill. The dead included the newly appointed Dr John Pierse; he was praised for his 'Herculean work' during the epidemic. Among the other victims that week were James Byrne, a farmer from Askintycloe, Ballindaggin, and a father and son, Patrick and Joseph Bolger of Patrick Street, Enniscorthy. A forcible entry was made into their house as neither had been seen out for some days. A resolution from the Galway BOG calling for the release of interned doctors to permit them to work during the influenza plague was rejected by the Wexford BOG but supported by the more nationalist Enniscorthy and Gorey BOGs.[80]

As the second wave started to subside in urban areas in mid-November, it continued to find fresh victims in rural Ireland. In mid-December, the Bunclody notes of the *Enniscorthy Guardian* reported the harrowing story of three young children dying in one family on the same day; as their coffins were placed in the hearse an ambulance came to take their father, mother and the rest of the grief stricken family to hospital.[81]

A third wave?

Towards the end of January, newspapers had a cautious tone of optimism that things were improving in the aftermath of the war and the influenza epidemic. The newly elected members of the first Dáil Éireann met for the opening session. The 1918 all-Ireland senior hurling final between Limerick and Wexford, deferred because of the epidemic in the autumn, eventually took place on Sunday, 26 January 1919. Wexford were beaten, but their senior football team had eventually beaten Louth in the deferred Leinster final that had been held the previous Sunday, 19 January. Wexford beat Tipperary in the all-Ireland football final on 16 February, winning a record four-in-row titles which still stands; Davy Tobin, Tipperary's top point scorer, had influenza and did not play.[82]

The optimism that things were improving in the aftermath of the influenza epidemic was misplaced. The Spanish flu re-emerged in a third wave in mid-February, in almost as aggressive a form as that in the autumn which had wreaked such havoc. In Dublin, the municipal public libraries were again closed by the public health authorities from Saturday, 1 March. At the Dublin Children's (Street Trading) Court the attendance was so low that the constables responsible for serving the summonses explained that in almost every house they visited there were one or more members of the families lying with influenza. Adjourning these cases, Alderman J.J. Kelly, JP, remarked that it was obvious that the number of sufferers among the very poor was exceptionally high.[83] The obituary columns of the *Irish Independent* on 3 March carried more death notices than on any given day during the previous wave. In the same paper, it was reported that claims for benefit from the Transport Workers' Union had increased from a norm of forty-three per week to more than eighty-five in the last week. Four members were reported dead on Saturday, in one case a man and his wife leaving a young family. The exceptional outbreak in the Celbridge district was reported as abating. In many parts of the country, two or more members of the same families were reported dead. The *Irish Times* recorded the inquest of Mrs Frances Phelan, aged twenty-seven, who lived with her husband, child and sister-in-law on Corporation Street, Dublin. Neighbours noticed the Phelans had not been seen for some time. The caretaker of the Corporation Buildings, John Maguire, said that when he entered, he found the four occupants of the room in the one bed, the baby with a comforter in its mouth, and Mrs Phelan already dead. He tried to rouse her husband and helped him to dress. The second woman, her sister-in-law, was partly dressed. He wrapped a coat about her, placed her on a chair, and sent a message to the police. The three were removed to Dublin Union Hospital by ambulance, but did not recover. John Irwin, a LGB official, complained to the inquest that named Union officials had been negligent in tending to the case, as it took some time for the ambulance to come; his complaint was denied by all the Union officials named.[84] Medical doctors reported that the dispensaries were under siege with influenza sufferers, and called for the closure of schools, theatres, churches and other places of assembly. Staff at Glasnevin Cemetery were being paid double time to work on Sundays because there were so many bodies awaiting burial.[85]

Charles Cameron wrote to the Lord Mayor of Dublin on 3 March suggesting that the Mansion House be closed to public assemblies; he mentioned there had been 143 deaths registered in Dublin from influenza in the week just ended, an increase of sixty-three compared with the previous one, but he was convinced the epidemic was declining.[86] Again, Cameron was trying to assuage public fear about the disease. However, the same newspaper which carried Cameron's letter also reported that there had been 335 burials in Glasnevin Cemetery alone the previous week; the discrepancy between the official numbers of deaths registered for influenza and the numbers buried at Glasnevin, which in non-epidemic situations would have expected twelve burials a day, as reported above, suggests that many influenza deaths are not included in the official statistics. The infant mortality was described by the newspaper as appalling. The number of burials of children under the age of two years often amounted to twenty-five a day. Glasnevin Cemetery burial records for March 1919 show 1,192 burials, compared to 593 in March 1918. The records also show page after page of child deaths.[87]

Outside Dublin, the disease continued to spread. The authorities in Belfast had reported that the epidemic there did not seem as virulent as in the autumn, its doctors and nurses were working day and night to attend to cases of influenza. Most of the primary schools were closed and preventative measures had been put in place in the secondary institutions. The tramcars, picture houses and places of entertainment had been disinfected. Baillie, the city's MOH, professed he was reluctant to order the closure of these places, as loss of income would make people more prone to the disease. In Co. Cork, Skibbereen Union, Adrigole and Rossmacowan parishes were also experiencing a widespread but not usually fatal outbreak.

Several deaths were reported in Clonakilty, according to the *Irish Independent*.[88] On Wednesday 5 March, the newspapers reported that more than seventy members of the DMP were off duty because of sickness, but so far only one of them had died. The burial orders for Glasnevin had reached eighty-two days before – the largest in the present outbreak; the previous day, there were fifty orders although the actual number of burials was seventy-nine.[89] In Athlone, so many corpses were waiting to be buried that hearses were unavailable on Sunday, and coffins had to be brought to the graveyard on outside cars and motorcars. In Belfast, places of amusement have been placed out of bounds to all ranks of navy and army, and to children aged up to fourteen years.

In the beginning of March five of the eleven political prisoners in Durham jail were reported to be suffering from the flu. Arthur Griffith sent a message home that relatives of the ten men in Gloucester jail who were suffering from influenza should not be alarmed.[90] Darrell Figgis, home on parole from Durham, reported that many of the prisoners were weakened by their long confinement; the flu's latest victims there had seemed to him to be the fittest of the lot and he feared for the others. They were, he said, fed the same food as the convicts, and their cells were like icehouses. He said that the internees' detention was unjustified, and called for their immediate release.[91] Figgis was known to embroider his stories.

Influenza claimed a second victim from the ranks of the Sinn Féin internees in Britain. Pierce McCan, a farmer, conscription activist and Sinn Féin Member of Parliament (MP) for Tipperary East, died on 6 March. As some of the Dublin daily newspapers eulogised the latest addition to the Sinn Féin martyrology, they also were enthused by the release of most of the internees. Several of those released were reported to be unfit to travel because of the effects of influenza, especially those detained in Durham. Arthur Griffith in Gloucester was reported as looking far from well. One of the internees revealed that the flu had never reached the internees in Reading, where many of the leaders of the Sinn Féin groups had been isolated.[92]

As the newspapers remarked on the subsidence of the epidemic in Dublin, seven more Irish internees who had been released from Gloucester jail but detained in hospital there suffering from influenza, returned home on 14 March. They were Séan MacEntee, MP, P. O'Keefe, MP, Thomas Hunter, MP, Dr Dillon, Frank Doran, J.J. O'Connell and P. Manahan. The Kildare MP Art O'Connor, in Durham, was still too ill to travel. Sir Charles Cameron said that although the epidemic was declining schools should remain closed until the week's death statistics were available. The pragmatic Cameron was correct; the Spanish lady's devastating tour of Ireland was coming, at last, to an end.[93]

Apart from the information it imparts about the epidemic itself, this survey of the influenza epidemic in the Dublin daily and regional weekly press raises two interesting issues. First of all, given that news coverage is usually driven by public interest, it seems that there was a regional variation in the interest level in the disease, and this variation was more evident in 1918, before the flu had spread extensively. The Dublin-based newspapers and those in Kildare, Louth, Carlow, Kilkenny and Wexford gave comprehensive coverage to the arrival and passage of the influenza, and recorded most aspects of it. The areas these newspapers covered were broadly similar to the areas which the official statistics show were most affected by the epidemic in 1918, indicating that the local experience of the influenza drove the amount of coverage in each newspaper. The second issue is that criticism of the Government's handling of or perceived failure to handle the crisis came from all sections of the press, not just from the pro-nationalist papers, an interesting observation at a time when newspapers' political allegiances were severely polarised, reflecting the political situation and the political allegiances of their readership. It was a time when the pro-establishment press might have been expected to be loyal to their own, refraining from criticism of the under-siege establishment. Even the archly pro-establishment *Irish Times* and the *Church of Ireland Gazette* expressed their displeasure at the way the LGB chose to handle the influenza crisis. The severity of local outbreaks of the influenza overcame the traditionally stronger political polarisation of some regional newspapers. This was particularly true in Naas, which was a black spot for influenza in late 1918. Some of the most incisive reporting of the epidemic comes from a 'Castle' paper, the *Kildare Observer*, whose coverage was highly critical of the authorities during the influenza crisis. Its competitor, the usually pro-nationalist *Leinster Leader*, also covered the flu extensively and fairly, its criticisms against the LGB not obviously founded in a desire to further the propagandist aims of the advanced nationalists, but in a desire to manage the influenza epidemic with due care. Other nationalist newspapers did use material of an advanced-nationalist type in connection with the epidemic (see Chapter 8).

This survey of the pandemic through the lens of the press shows how the pandemic pushed war and other news back as it passed through towns and local communities, silencing activities as people took to their sick beds. It reveals a high level of public awareness about the effects of the Spanish influenza pandemic both on the island of Ireland and in other parts of the world. The fact that this awareness existed, that regional and national newspapers were carrying warnings of its arrival and detailing its effects on the populace, begs some questions: why was a disease that dominated the columns of newspapers, was so immersed in the popular psyche, connected to the growing nationalism, a disease which was part of a big international story, left out of Irish historiography for almost 100 years?

Notes

1 Felix M. Larkin, *Irish Independent*, 16 February 2016.
2 J.E. Doherty and D.J. Hickey, *A Chronology of Irish History Since 1500* (Dublin:Gill and Macmillan, 1989), p. 188.
3 *Irish Independent*, 1 June 1918.
4 *Irish Independent*, 3 June 1918.
5 *Irish Independent*, 4 June 1918.
6 *Annual report of the chief medical officer, 1919–1920* (1920), xvii, cmd 978; the author attributes the smallpox reference to Prinzing's *Epidemics resulting from Wars*. See also, for example, *Irish Times*, 31 October 1918.
7 *Belfast Newsletter*, 11 June 1918.
8 *Irish Independent*, 20 June 1918.
9 *Midland Reporter and Westmeath Nationalist*, 20 June 1918.
10 *Irish Independent*, 24 June 1918.
11 *Irish Independent*, 25 June 1918.
12 *Irish Independent*, 26 June 1918.
13 For more on Cameron, see Lydia Carroll, *In the Fever King's Preserves; Sir Charles Cameron and the Dublin Slums* (Dublin: A & A Farmar, 2011).
14 *Irish Independent*, 26 June 1918.
15 See the World Health Organization fact sheet on plague www.who.int/mediacentre/factsheets/fs267/en/ (accessed 12 June 2017).
16 *Irish Independent*, 4 July 1918.
17 *Irish Independent*, 4 July 1918.
18 *Midland Reporter and Westmeath Nationalist*, 11 July 1918.
19 *Evening Herald*, 3 and 4 October 1918.
20 *Evening Herald*, 7 October 1918.
21 *Evening Herald*, 10 October 1918.
22 *Irish Times*, 11 October 1918.
23 *Irish Independent*, 16 October 1918.
24 *Irish Independent*, 16 October 1918.
25 *Evening Herald*, 16 October 1918.
26 *Evening Herald*, 17 October 1918.
27 *Irish Times*, 17 October 1918.
28 *Wicklow People*, 19 October 1918.

29 *Wicklow People*, 19 October 1918.
30 *Wicklow People*, 26 October 1918.
31 *Irish Times* and *Irish Independent*, 18 October 1918.
32 *Irish Independent*, 24 October 1918.
33 *Evening Herald*, 19 and 21 October 1918.
34 *Irish Independent*, 23 October 1918.
35 *Irish Independent*, 4 March 1919.
36 *Evening Herald*, 23 and 24 October 1918.
37 *Evening Herald*, 29 October 1918.
38 *Evening Herald*, 29 October 1918.
39 *Evening Herald*, 26 October 1918.
40 *Irish Independent*, 28 October 1918.
41 *Irish Independent*, 6 November 1918.
42 *Irish Times*, 31 October 1918.
43 *Irish Independent* and *Evening Herald*, 10 December 1918.
44 *Irish Independent*, 24 January 1919.
45 *Kildare Observer*, 19 October 1918.
46 *Kildare Observer*, 26 October 1918.
47 *Kildare Observer*, 26 October 1918.
48 *Kildare Observer*, 26 October 1918.
49 *Kildare Observer*, 2 November 1918.
50 *Kildare Observer*, 26 October and 2 November 1918.
51 *Kildare Observer*, 2 November 1918.
52 *Kildare Observer*, 23 November 1918.
53 *Kildare Observer*, 26 October 1918.
54 *Kildare Observer*, 9 November 1918.
55 *Kildare Observer*, 30 November 1918.
56 *Dundalk Democrat and People's Journal*, 26 October 1918.
57 Ibid.
58 *Dundalk Democrat and People's Journal*, 26 October 1918. The Custom House was the office of the LGB. It was burned during the revolutionary period, its records deliberately destroyed.
59 Ibid.
60 Ibid.
61 *Dundalk Democrat*, 9 November 1918.
62 *Dundalk Democrat*, 16 November 1918.
63 *Dundalk Democrat*, 16 and 23 November 1918.
64 *Kilkenny People*, 19 October 1918.
65 *Kilkenny People*, 26 October 1918.
66 *Kilkenny People*, 2 November 1918.
67 *Kilkenny People*, 2 November 1918.
68 *Kilkenny People*, 9 November 1918.

69 *Kilkenny People*, 16 November 1918.

70 *Kilkenny People*, 23 November 1918

71 *Enniscorthy Guardian*, 19 October 1918.

72 *Enniscorthy Guardian*, 26 October 1918.

73 *The People*, 31 October 1918.

74 *Enniscorthy Guardian*, 2 November 1918.

75 *The People*, 2 November 1918.

76 *Enniscorthy Guardian*, 9 November 1918.

77 *Enniscorthy Guardian*, 16 November 1918.

78 *Enniscorthy Guardian*, 16 November 1918.

79 Mr Doran's two brothers-in-law, who worked as shop assistants in Arklow, also died during the epidemic. See interview with Lena Higgins, Chapter 7.

80 *Enniscorthy Guardian* and *the People*, 23 November 1918.

81 *Enniscorthy Guardian*, 14 December 1918.

82 *Irish Independent*, 26 January 1919.

83 *Irish Independent*, 3 March 1919.

84 *Irish Times*, 26 February 1919; *Weekly Irish Times*, 1 March 1919.

85 *Weekly Irish Times*, 1 March 1919.

86 *Irish Independent*, 4 March 1919.

87 Glasnevin Cemetery burial records, kindly supplied by Conor Dodd and Georgina Laragy.

88 *Irish Independent*, 4 March 1919.

89 *Irish Independent*, 5 March 1919.

90 *Irish Independent*, 3 March 1919.

91 *Irish Independent*, 3 March 1919.

92 *Irish Independent*, 7 and 8 March 1919. For a further discussion of influenza among the 'German' plot internees, see Chapter 8.

93 *Midland Reporter and Westmeath Nationalist*, 3 April 1919.

3

Counting the ill and the dead

'How many died?' is usually the first question asked about the pandemic. The answer is not straightforward, for two main reasons: difficulty of influenza diagnosis, and the sheer numbers dying in concentrated periods during the three waves. Doctors focused on keeping those still living alive, rather than certifying deaths. There is also the added complication that the numbers dying from infectious diseases had been reducing noticeably since the beginning of the decade. This chapter aims to unravel some of the complexities of counting the Irish dead from the pandemic, beginning with a brief explanatory history of the development of disease death statistics.

Developing national death statistics

When a series of epidemics caused chaos in the nineteenth century, twelve nations took part in seven sanitary conferences in Paris, Vienna, Washington, Rome and Constantinople between 1851 and 1892 to negotiate international monitoring of cholera, plague and yellow fever; they reached a limited accord, but the impetus was positive. By 1907, the co-operation had developed into work that was to have real merit in combatting outbreaks of epidemic disease, with the establishment of a permanent organisation to monitor international levels of certain diseases, the Office International d'Hygiène Publique (OIHP), located in Paris. It received notification of serious communicable diseases from the twenty-three participating nations, retransmitting this information to the member nations, and developed sanitary conventions and quarantine regulations on shipping and train travel. This organisation was later absorbed into the World Health Organization (WHO) in 1948.[1]

Britain and Ireland were part of this international trend towards improving and standardising health systems. Monitoring systems had been pioneered in England and Wales by the English medical statistician, William Farr, compiler of the abstracts in the English RG's department, and as a result England (together with Wales) was considered the first sanitary nation. Registration of births, marriages and deaths became compulsory in England and Wales in 1836. Farr developed a disease classification which enabled him to analyse mortality and morbidity statistics, as he recognised that such monitoring of the population's health could lead to real improvements.[2] In Ireland, the polymath William Wilde - then a precocious twenty-six-year old - was invited by the census commissioners to write on the causes of death for the 1841 census, in the wake of the introduction of death registration in England and Wales - which permitted him to analyse the 1832–33 cholera epidemic. Wilde's work on this census established disease rubrics of classification; he was subsequently involved more closely, through formal appointment as an assistant census commissioner with developing statistical analysis of disease in the censuses of 1851, 1861 and 1871.[3] Ireland's first annual report of births, deaths and marriages was compiled for the year 1864.

Farr's classification was adopted, with amendments, by the International Statistical Congress in 1864; it was again revised by Jacques Bertillon. The ISC's successor, the International Statistical Institute, called for the adoption of Bertillon's revisions by all European statistical institutions in 1900, following its adoption in North America, most of South America and many European countries.[4] This International List of Causes of Death (ICD) was to become a major tool in the compilation of statistics on the 1918–19 influenza pandemic in these islands, as it had been adopted by the RGs of Ireland, England and Wales, and of Scotland, to classify certified deaths in their annual vital statistics reports.

Standardising the classification of death was intended to enable more accurate international comparison of causes of death, but difficulties of definition remained for many years, and diseases would be reclassified in the light of newer scientific understanding. This list is still revisited at intervals of about ten years, incorporating any necessary changes. The classification system groups disease and morbid conditions into associated clusters, with the attribution of a number to individual diseases.[5] The standard used during the influenza pandemic was the 1911 revision of the ICD; the Irish RG's reports for 1918–19 show that it defined 189 possible causes of death, with some further sub-classification. Influenza was clustered with epidemic diseases, whereas different types of pneumonia were clustered with other lung diseases.

The diagnosis of influenza and decisions on causes of death during influenza epidemics pose quite a difficulty for investigators. Influenza is notoriously difficult to diagnose definitively, as its symptoms resemble those of many other infective diseases; even today, doctors will insist on a diagnosis of influenza-like illness until a case is confirmed by laboratory testing. Leo van Bergen has observed that many people diagnosed in 1918–19 as having died of tuberculosis, bronchitis, heart failure, malaria, cholera, dysentery, measles or typhus probably actually died of flu, whether or not their health was compromised by other health problems. At the initial stages of the epidemic, influenza was more likely to be confused with other diseases with similar symptoms, particularly as the first wave occurred out of season. Once the flu became known, misdiagnosis occurred in the other direction as well.[6] The ICD was arranged so that only one cause of death was possible; this issue proved problematic to the registration of some dual-cause deaths during the pandemic. Did they die from influenza, or from the frequent complication of pneumonia, heart failure or other causes? The list was subsequently revised to permit the listing of all influenza deaths with complicating pneumonias in a separate grouping. That left a recognised problem of what to do with deaths from other sequelae of influenza. Ought they be attributed to the sequela or to the influenza?[7]

Improving health

Throughout the latter part of the nineteenth century Irish local authorities (who answered to the LGB, which also bore overall responsibility for the Poor Law dispensary network introduced under the 1851 Medical Charities Act) had made a series of improvements in public sanitation which were reflected in improving health statistics. Dublin Corporation had, since the 1860s, established a disinfection depot at Marrowbone Lane, a rudimentary sewage treatment system,

an abattoir, an isolation hospital, a sanatorium for treating tuberculosis, and a municipal laboratory. In 1879, the city's rate of death
from infectious diseases was nine per thousand of living population;
by 1919, it had been reduced to 1.3 per thousand. Typhus deaths had
been reduced from 170 in 1881 to none for three years from 1916 to
1919, according to the city's executive sanitary officer and medical
superintendent of health, Sir Charles Cameron.[8] Cameron's opinion
was shared by the RG, Sir William J. Thompson, who reported to
parliament in 1920 that the years 1918–19 would have been record
years for low mortality from all causes in Ireland, were it not for the
excessive deaths from pneumonia and influenza.[9] In January 1918,
Thompson told the Royal Academy of Medicine in Ireland that mortality from disease had shown a marked decrease in Ireland, as in
England and Wales and Scotland over the previous fifty years. Irish
mortality from tuberculosis in the period 1911–15 had decreased by 13
per cent compared with 1866–70, and infant mortality had decreased
by 4 per cent compared with the same period. Infant mortality in
Ireland in 1911–15 was 21 per cent under that of England and Wales,
and some 24 per cent under that for Scotland.[10] These figures and
opinions indicate that the overall health of Ireland's population was
not unreasonable by European standards when the influenza pandemic arrived on its shores, and that even the health of Dubliners –
where many were housed in atrocious conditions – was improving.
They offer evidence that Irish health was improving in line with the
epidemiological transition theory first posited by Abdel Omran in
1971 to describe the decline of mortality from infectious diseases due
to a complex fusion of environmental, demographic, economic and
sociologic as well as medical determinants.[11]

Influenza mortality

Statisticians at the Irish General Register Office (GRO) rigorously
examined data collated during the three waves of the pandemic. The
RG Sir William Thompson gave it careful and detailed consideration
in his annual reports, and read a paper on it to the Statistical and
Social Inquiry Society of Ireland on 14 November 1918, which was
later printed in the society's journal with the title 'Mortality from
influenza in Ireland'; this was subsequently printed in full in the
Dublin Journal of Medical Science.[12]

In Thompson's opinion, the outstanding feature of mortality statistics for 1918 and 1919 was not just the deaths from flu, but also pneumonia, a frequent complication partly responsible for the high fatality rate of the pandemic. In 1918, there were reportedly 10,651 influenza deaths on the island, compared to an average for the previous ten years of 1,234 influenza deaths. There were 6,120 deaths from pneumonia, compared to an average of 4,067 for the previous ten years, and a 50 per cent increase on the previous year.[13] The death rate from influenza per thousand of living population over the entire year was 2.43; the death rate from pneumonia was 1.4, compared to an average of 0.93 for the preceding ten years. There were 9,406 influenza deaths in 1919, and 5,245 deaths from pneumonia, an annual death rate of 2.11 per thousand of living population for influenza and 1.18 for pneumonia.[14] Hence, the reports total 20,057 influenza deaths; by adding the 3,231 total excess deaths from pneumonia to the total for influenza, the death toll caused by the influenza epidemic increased to 23,288. Other figures for the death toll from influenza in Ireland have been offered. Edwin Oakes Jordan included an Irish estimate of 18,367 in the first estimate of global mortality, but his estimate was based on a figure Thompson had given for the twelve months of 1918 and the first quarter of 1919, which obviously did not include low levels of influenza still occurring after the peak waves had passed.[15] Niall Johnston took this figure from Jordan to compile his estimate of global mortality.[16] Aside from pneumonia, deaths caused by influenza may, as indicated above, have been attributed to other diseases, but against the background of decreasing mortality from all causes it is difficult to measure this in an Irish context.[17] Graphing deaths from bronchitis in 1918 and 1919 with deaths from influenza and pneumonia showed little evidence of a correlation, perhaps because the influenza pandemic was masking a background decrease in deaths certified to bronchitis. Bronchitis was still a significant killer, causing over 7 per cent of all deaths, but at 5,794 deaths, the 1918 total was 770 below that for 1917 and 1,046 below the ten-year average. The RG's report for 1920 mentions a 'considerable reduction' in the number of deaths from bronchitis in that year, falling from 6,593 in 1919 to 5,241 in 1920.[18] The numbers dying from heart disease in 1918 amounted to almost 9 per cent of the deaths recorded, but were 1,225 below the average for the previous ten years.

Infection estimates

Statistics for epidemic disease tend to focus on the dead rather than on the survivors. Historians of Spanish flu have tended to concentrate on the mortality statistics, their first gaze entranced by the millions of dead and the speed with which the disease spread around the globe. Time and the death statistics have acted as fences in a fog, obscuring from them the real statistical story of the influenza: the exceptional levels of morbidity. The disease was not particularly lethal; international statisticians and historians often use a death rate of 2.5 per cent of those who actually caught the disease (case fatality rate) to estimate morbidity.[19] Applying this rate to the official estimation of Irish influenza dead, 20,057 would give a morbidity of approximately 800,000, or about one fifth of the island's population at the time. By taking the excess dead from pneumonia into the equation, we can estimate with reasonable authority that over 900,000 people caught this strain of influenza.

Mortality from the influenza pandemic of 1918–19 was concentrated in most parts of the world in three waves, each lasting several weeks, the first in spring or early summer of 1918, the second wave, which usually caused higher levels of morbidity and therefore mortality, in the autumn and winter of 1918, and the third in the spring of 1919. In some areas, a fourth wave occurred, usually in 1920.[20] The Irish experience of influenza followed this three wave international pattern. The waves occurred in June–July 1918, from mid-October to December 1918, and from mid-February to mid-April 1919. Figure 1 charts the occurrence of these waves of influenza and the correlating waves of pneumonia in the Dublin registration area over an eighteen-month period.

Thompson tabulated the annual influenza and pneumonia mortality statistics by province, county and age period in the 1918 and 1919 reports, and estimated the death rates per estimated thousand living. Using Thompson's influenza tables to establish the provincial mortality from influenza, it becomes apparent that Ulster and Leinster had many more influenza deaths than either Munster or Connacht (see Figure 2). Ulster suffered the higher total numbers, with 4,773 deaths in 1918 and 2,809 in 1919, out of a population in the 1911 census of 1,581,696. Leinster, the second most populated province with 1,162,044 in 1911, had 3,535 deaths in 1918 and 2,588

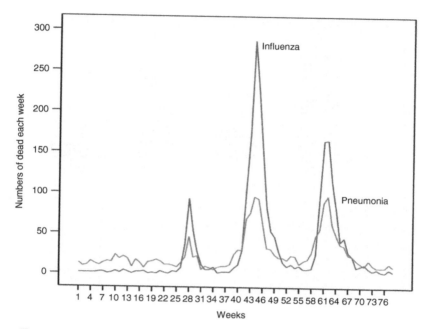

Figure 1 Weekly deaths from influenza and pneumonia in the Dublin registration area, January 1918 – June 1919.

(Source: weekly returns of births, deaths and marriages of the registrar general.)

in 1919. Munster, with a population in 1911 of 1,035,495, lost 1,646 to the disease in 1918 and 2,187 in 1919, as the epidemic moved westward from the east coast. Like Munster, Connacht fared worse in the third wave than in the first two, although the difference was more dramatic. With a 1911 population of 610,984, it had 697 influenza victims in 1918; the total more than doubled in 1919, to 1,822 (see Figure 2).

Ulster, with the highest population base of the four provinces, had 1,459 more influenza deaths than its closest contender for the dubious title of interprovincial influenza champion, Leinster. By using Thompson's death rates instead of a simple numerical total to measure the scale of the problem in each province, it is possible to reverse the position of Leinster and Ulster (see Figure 3). The constant high volume of human traffic through Dublin and other east coast ports – Dundalk, Howth and Wexford – to Britain probably

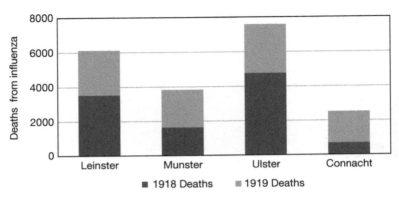

Figure 2 Influenza deaths in each province in 1918 and 1919.
(Source: annual reports of the registrar general for Ireland.)

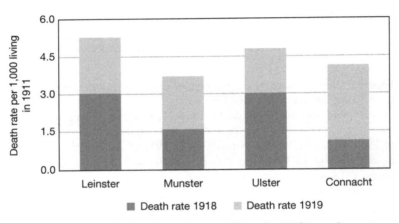

Figure 3 Influenza death rate per thousand living (in 1911) in each province.
(Source: annual reports of the registrar general for Ireland.)

played a major part in accounting for Leinster's higher death rate.
High levels of urbanisation, with workers in close contact in large
factories, probably contributed to Ulster's death rate.[21] The reason for
Connacht's higher influenza death rate of 2.98 per thousand of living
population in 1919 is not clear, but it has been speculated that it could
have something to do with seasonal labour movements, particularly
in Mayo, which are associated with the planting of tillage crops.

Figures 4 and 5 confirm newspaper reports that north-east Ulster and eastern Leinster bore the brunt of the first and second waves – entering through ports like Belfast, Dundalk, Howth and Dublin and spreading first through local urban populations – and seems to suggest that the influenza epidemic effectively moved westward in the third wave. The highest death rates from influenza in 1918, measured per thousand of living population in 1911 (the census year), were in Carlow, Dublin, Kildare, Wicklow and Wexford, Armagh, Belfast, Donegal, Down and Monaghan.

More people died in Co. Kildare, at 3.95 per thousand of living population, than in any other county. Kildare's exceptionally high rate of death from influenza in 1918 may have been partly attributable to local factors in Naas, where water and power shortages caused added hardship at the height of the second wave.[22] Naas accounted for 144 of the county total of 265 influenza deaths in 1918. While the return of soldiers from the arena of war has been suggested as an explanation for this exceptional county rate, arguments that complicate this are presented in Chapter 4. Local historian Frank Taaffe has suggested that the early outbreak in Athy could be traced to workers coming from Belfast to work on the railway.[23] The county's strong social and rail links with Dublin must also have played a role, and the local conditions in Naas mentioned in the previous chapter.

The lowest county influenza death rate in 1918 was in Co. Clare, with only forty-nine deaths and a rate of 0.46 per thousand of living population. The county's infamously poor rail infrastructure, pilloried in the Percy French song 'Are you right there, Michael', may have actually helped it escape the worst ravages of the influenza crisis through social distancing.[24] Other western counties, Leitrim and Mayo had a very low incidence of influenza in 1918 also. In 1919, the highest rates were in Longford (3.04), Mayo (the highest at 3.27) and Donegal (3.26).

Seasonal migration and the location of a British naval base at Lough Swilly were probably the major factors behind Donegal's unusually high incidence of influenza in both years, spanning all three waves. Donegal had a tradition of providing seasonal agricultural labour; Patricia Marsh has suggested that Donegal migrant labourers or emigrants to Scotland who brought influenza victims' bodies for burial in their native county, by boat, may have spread the infection. The presence of a naval base in Rathmullan may also have been a factor in the repeated reintroduction of infection. Although the US naval base had hospital ship facilities in Cork (which may have prevented the continual reintroduction of infection into local communities), navy and army personnel in Donegal were treated in local hospitals, which also contributed to the spread of infection.[25] The lowest rate of influenza mortality in 1919 was in Belfast, with a rate of 0.79 deaths per thousand of living population. Figures 4 and 5 use Thompson's influenza tables to map influenza death rates by county in 1918 and 1919. They show the influenza's sweep across the country in an approximate east–west direction over the two years, with exceptions for local circumstances such as Donegal and Dublin. Outside the two largest cities, Dublin and Belfast, Ireland has essentially a rural population, with an even scattering of market towns or less populous cities in each county. It is worth noting that Donegal and Kildare – and Mayo in 1919 – essentially rural populations with only small towns, have rates of death that compare with those of the bigger cities, Dublin and Belfast. So although city living conditions clearly exacerbated the influenza issues, rural areas were also badly affected.

Some authorities have made the argument that mortality from Spanish influenza was gendered; they describe the flu as appearing to target young, previously healthy males. The Irish data shows an almost even gender distribution, with slightly more males than females in both years (53 per cent of all flu deaths were male).

Figure 6 charts the influenza deaths in Leinster by age group and numbers of dead.[26] It shows the higher mortality from influenza in the under-five age group, and in the young adult sector. Figure 7 shows a similar pattern for the total registered Irish mortality from influenza by age group. These graphs show that the Irish mortality from influenza followed the international pattern with mortality peaking in the mid-life period, between the ages of twenty-five and thirty-four. The graph also shows that the flu killed disproportionately in the twenty–forty-four-year-old sector. The scale of death from this sector of society represented in this chart must have left large numbers of children without at least one parent, and families struggling to survive. Figure 8 plots the death rates in each year in each age group per thousand of living population and reveals that the real damage the influenza did in 1918 was to the twenty–thirty-four-year age group. It also emphasises that children under the age of five were far more

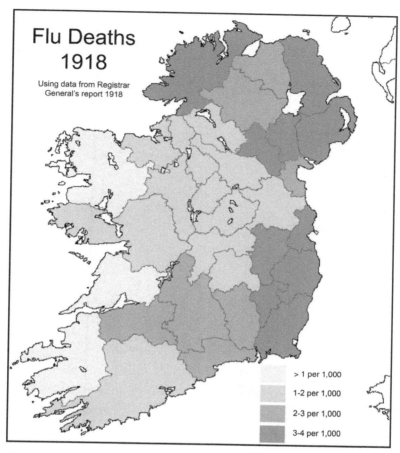

Flu Deaths 1918

Using data from Registrar General's report 1918

> 1 per 1,000
1-2 per 1,000
2-3 per 1,000
3-4 per 1,000

Figure 4 Map of influenza deaths by county in 1918. Statistics from the annual reports of the registrar general. Deaths expressed in death rate per thousand living.

likely, in proportion to the numbers living in their group, to die from influenza than their older siblings. Children aged from five to fourteen years experienced the lowest rates of death in any age group. The closure of schools may have played a role in preventing death in this age sector, while another factor may simply have been that children, unlike their working parents, could stay in bed when they became ill, as doctors recommended throughout the epidemic.

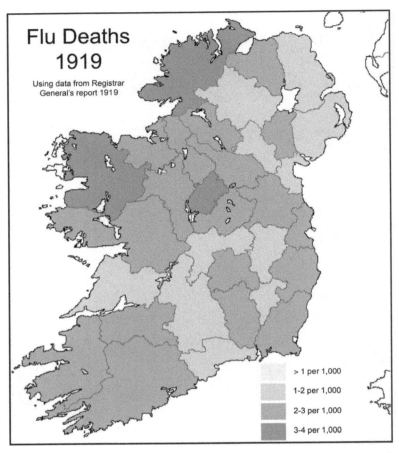

Flu Deaths 1919

Using data from Registrar General's report 1919

> 1 per 1,000
1-2 per 1,000
2-3 per 1,000
3-4 per 1,000

Figure 5 Map of influenza deaths by county in 1919. Statistics from the annual reports of the registrar general. Deaths expressed in death rate per thousand living.

Influenza is now generally recognised as being more likely to cause severe illness in pregnant women than in women who are not pregnant, and pregnant women in many countries, including Ireland are advised to have the influenza vaccination. The US Center for Disease Control's influenza information web pages explains that changes in the immune system, heart and lungs during pregnancy make pregnant women (and women up to two weeks post-partum)

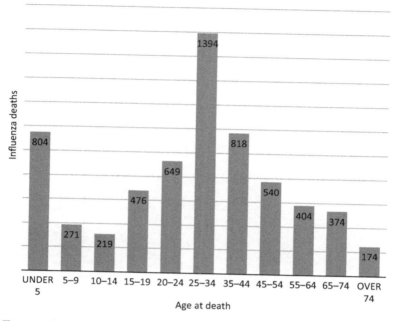

Figure 6 Influenza deaths in Leinster by age group, 1918–19.
(Source: annual returns of the registrar general, 1918–19.)

more prone to severe illness from flu, as well as to hospitalisations and even death. Pregnant women with flu also have a greater chance for serious problems for their developing baby, including premature labour and delivery.[27] Some 266 deaths or 2.9 per cent of the total recorded female influenza deaths in Scotland in 1918–19 were from diseases or accidents of pregnancy associated with influenza.[28] In Ireland in 1918, 5060 women are certified as dying from influenza. Twenty-six were pregnant; another fifteen pregnant women died from pneumonia. Some 509 women died during pregnancy from all causes in 1918. In 1919, 4,485 women were certified to have died from influenza. Fifty-three of the 524 pregnant women who died in 1919 were victims of influenza, six were victims of pneumonia. Fifty-two of these were aged between twenty and forty-four out of a total of 1,680 female deaths in the same age group, or 3.2 per cent of the influenza deaths in this age group. Over the two years, almost 10 per cent of the recorded deaths of pregnant women were

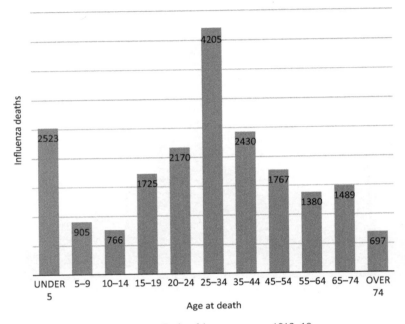

Figure 7 Influenza deaths in Ireland by age group, 1918–19.
(Source: annual returns of the registrar general, 1918–19.)

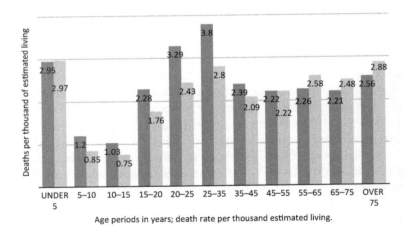

Figure 8 Death rates from influenza in Ireland at each age period in 1918 and 1919.
(Source: annual returns of the registrar general, 1918–19.)

caused by either influenza or pneumonia. This total represented less than 1 per cent of the total recorded female deaths from influenza, a statistically insignificant rate when compared to the equivalent Scottish rate of 2.9 per cent of the total.[29]

Death by social class and occupation

The weekly returns of the RG for the Dublin registration area provide insights into the burden each class and class sector suffered. Figure 9 draws on these weekly reports to give deaths by social class or occupation in the Dublin registration area during the period covering the peak three waves of the epidemic, while Figure 10 compares these death rates per thousand of living population. The Class 1 sector – which included medical doctors, clergy, lawyers, army and naval officers, and higher civil servants as well as the propertied classes and higher class merchants and manufacturers – was, with 14,658 members, proportionately much smaller than any

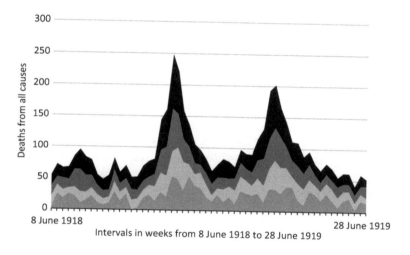

Figure 9 Deaths in Dublin by social class and occupation, June 1918 – June 1919.

(Source: weekly reports of the registrar general, 1918–19, using the class and occupation categories in the reports, where Class 1 is the professional and independent class, Class 2 the middle class, Class 3 the artisan class and petty shopkeepers and Class 4 the general service class.)

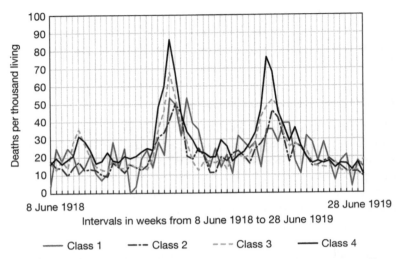

Figure 10 Death rate in Dublin by social class and occupation, June 1918 – June 1919, showing values for weekly death rates from all causes per thousand living.

(Source: weekly reports of the registrar general, 1918–19, using the class and occupation categories in the reports, where Class 1 is the professional and independent class, Class 2 the middle class, Class 3 the artisan class and petty shopkeepers and Class 4 the general service class.)

of the other three classes; it represented only 3.7 per cent of the total population of 397,957, based on 1911 census statistics. The middle-class group (Class 2) had 101,798 people in 1911, the artisan and petty shopkeepers (Class 3) had 108,420 and the general service class (Class 4) had 167,479 members, families of people who worked as domestic servants, hawkers, labourers, drivers, and in the prison, army, postal and police services.[30]

These class death statistics (Figure 9) indicate a surprisingly strong correlation over the thirteen-month period, suggesting that influenza was a socially neutral disease in relation to mortality.[31] This correlation was also broadly maintained in Figure 10, where the classes are compared by death per thousand of living population, using annualised weekly rates. The chart serves to indicate, however, that Class 3 and particularly Class 4 experienced higher death rates than the other two classes during the two more severe waves of the epidemic in Dublin, suggesting that there was an element of class dependency for mortality from this influenza.

Who was statistically most likely to die?

The collated weekly death statistics for Dublin for the fourth quarter of 1918, which conveniently includes the entire second wave of the influenza, confirm that high death rates from influenza were not so much class-dependent as job-dependent. They tally with newspaper reports (in Chapter 2) that indicate people who worked with the public – shop workers, police, medical workers, bank officials, priests – were more likely to catch and therefore more likely to die from a disease.

The annualised death rate in the families of the professional and independent classes in the final quarter of 1918 was 31.9 per thousand of living population in 1911, compared to 26.7 per thousand of living population in the middle classes, 29.7 in the artisan class and petty shopkeepers' category, and 38.5 in the general service class. Within each of these class categories the RG made between three and six subdivisions. It is quite clear from the death rates in these subdivisions that occupations which involved dealing with the public carried a high risk for the worker and their families. Within the professional class, the highest rates of deaths occurred in the clerical, medical, legal, military officers and other professions, representing an annual death rate of 52.4 per thousand of living population. Of these 103 deaths, forty-eight were in the twenty-five–forty-five age bracket, with four of the deaths attributed to pneumonia, four attributed to other diseases of the respiratory system, and seventy-four to 'other causes'. By contrast, higher class merchants and manufacturers had a death rate of only 5.9, and in the category for people of rank and property the death rate was eight per thousand living. In the middle-class category, the rate among banking and civil service officials was 24.8 per thousand living, and among business managers and traders apart from petty shopkeepers was 21.6; clerks and commercial assistants had a death rate of 32.8 per thousand living. Among the category for artisans and petty shopkeepers,[32] the highest rates were, perhaps surprisingly, not in the subdivisions for petty shopkeepers, at 28.4 per thousand living, but in a subdivision called 'other trades and callings ranking with trades' (plumbers for example), at 41.9 per thousand living.

The real disaster was in the general service class subdivision for the army, police, postal deliverers and prison services, workers who were constantly mingling with other people and therefore at greater risk of getting infected. Some 390 died in the fourth quarter, out of a 1911 population of 12,977, an annualised death rate of 120.2 per thousand of living population. Of these, seventy-seven were certified to pneumonia and twenty-two to other diseases of the respiratory system, and 215 to 'other causes'. Children under five accounted for 116 or 30 per cent of these deaths, while another 131 (34 per cent) were aged between twenty-five and forty-five. Domestic service was a comparatively safe occupation, with a death rate of 17.2 per thousand living. In the category for hawkers, porters and labourers, 959 died out of the 103,081 population in 1911, a rate of 37.2 per thousand living; once causes which were definitely not influenza were excluded, the possibility that 801 of these deaths might be connected to the pandemic emerges. A massive 315 of these were children under the age of five. Of the 493 who died in workhouses during the quarter, eighty-two were attributed to pneumonia, eighty-one to other diseases of the respiratory system, and 241 to 'other causes'.[33]

In the first quarter of 1919, the annualised death rate in the subdivision for clerical, medical, legal, military officers and heads of public departments was again high, at 41.2 per thousand living, compared with a rate of 27 per thousand living for the entire professional and independent class. The merchant and manufacturing subdivision had a rate of 3 per thousand living. In the 'artisans and petty shopkeepers' class, the subdivision 'other trades and callings ranking with trades' was again badly affected, having a rate of 43 per thousand living. The general service class subdivision for the army, police, postal deliverers and prison services had an annualised death rate of 96.7, with 292 deaths, of which 113 were children under five years of age, seventy-six were of adults aged from twenty-five to forty-four; forty-nine were certified as pneumonia and thirty-one as 'other respiratory disease', with 141 attributed to other causes. Of the 3,811 deaths in this quarter, 1,584 were in the general service class. Again, domestic service was a relatively safe haven, with only 149 of the 36,041 domestic servants and their families dying during the quarter, forty-nine from pneumonia and thirty-one from other respiratory diseases.

Nursing sick children may have made parents more prone to dying from influenza. The subdivision for hawkers, porters and labourers was the largest individual subdivision, with 103,081 people in 1911. Although the annualised death rate was not as shockingly high as among the army, police, postal services and prison services category at 39.3 per thousand living, the sheer size of the subdivision makes the number of dead in this quarter, at 1,014, seem formidable. Some 339, or almost 9 per cent of all Dublin deaths for the quarter, were of children in this subdivision under the age of five; 165 were adults aged twenty-five–forty-four, and 214 were adults aged forty-five–sixty-four. Many of these deaths can be laid squarely at the feet of the epidemic: 155 were certified to pneumonia, 191 to other respiratory disease, and 463 to 'other causes'.

A week of pandemic death in Dublin: November 1918

By examining the 562 deaths in a week at the height of the second wave of the pandemic – ending 2 November 1918 – we obtain a snapshot of which human lives the disease was taking, and see how difficult it can be for researchers of the pandemic to read cause-of-death tables.[34]

Figure 11 charts the deaths from all causes in the Dublin registration area that week. It shows that ninety-nine of the total

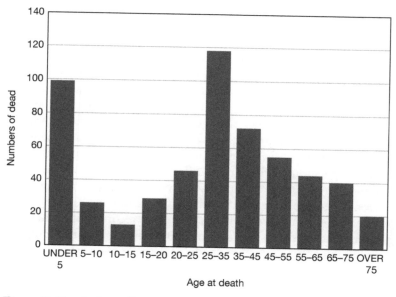

Figure 11 Deaths from all causes in Dublin in week ending 2 November 1918. (Source: all statistics derived from the weekly report of the registrar general, and refer to the Dublin registration area.)

562 deaths were children under five, who accounted for 17.6 per cent of the week's deaths. In the twenty-five–forty-four age group, there were 190 deaths, 33.8 per cent of the total deaths. These two groups, representing twenty-five years of life, had over 50 per cent of the deaths for the week. The RG's tables carry fixed categories of causes of death. These categories include the notifiable epidemic diseases, such as typhus, smallpox and measles, as well as tuberculosis, diarrhoea, convulsions, cancer and diseases of the respiratory system, subdivided into 'pneumonia' and 'other'; there was no category for influenza. Of the week's deaths, ninety-six were attributed to pneumonia, and thirty-seven to 'other respiratory diseases'. The vast majority of the deaths, 369 or 65.7 per cent, were attributed to 'other causes'. The RG's table highlights the difficulties faced by statisticians and historians trying to assess the damage the epidemic caused. By combining the deaths from diseases of the respiratory system (on the grounds that many diseases of the respiratory system, for example pneumonia and bronchitis, might actually have been caused by influenza) with 'other causes' the combined total of 502 represents 89.3 per cent of the deaths in the registration area during the week.

Another table in this weekly report does give a breakdown of the influenza-certified deaths by age in the Dublin registration area, but again, the data present puzzles for the researcher. Figure 12 charts 287 deaths certified to influenza for the week ending 2 November 1918; the equivalent week over the preceding decade had recorded an average of 0.8 influenza deaths. This chart shows again that children under the age of five and adults aged twenty-five–thirty-five were particularly vulnerable to the disease. Looking again at the under-fives deaths in Figures 11 and 12, the numbers in that age group dying from influenza seem low compared to the numbers dying from all causes. By referring back to the RG's tables, it becomes clear that many of the deaths in this age group may have been caused by influenza but were recorded as bronchitis, pneumonia, or febrile convulsions. Does this suggest that doctors were more likely to attribute deaths of younger children to respiratory diseases rather than to influenza? The same also appears to apply to deaths of over fifty-fives, but the numbers involved in that age group were much smaller. This is an important find, as it further supports the grounds to doubt the total deaths for the pandemic compiled by the RG. The real number, particularly in relation to the deaths of young children, could be much higher. The thirty-two deaths from bronchitis recorded that week were more than double the average for the equivalent week in the previous decade, which was 15.6. There were ninety-six recorded deaths from pneumonia compared to an average of 9.8 for the equivalent week over the preceding decade. The numbers of deaths from cerebral haemorrhage, heart disease, whooping cough and acute nephritis, all possible sequelae of influenza or misdiagnosis of influenza, also exceeded the average for the same week in the previous decennial. It must be remembered that theses excesses occurred in a year where deaths from all causes not associated with the influenza epidemic were falling. There were also marked increases in mortality from cancer, pulmonary tuberculosis, old age and congenital disability, which are worthy of note in the context of the peak mortality week of the influenza epidemic in the capital. A plausible suggestion for these increases might be that influenza sometimes reaped impending deaths from other causes (such as cancer, pulmonary tuberculosis and even old age) early.

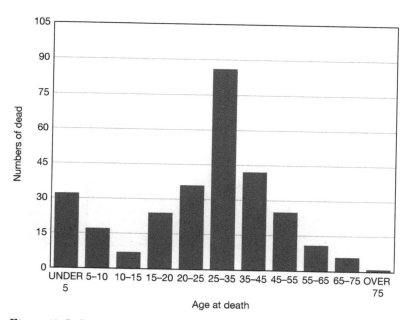

Figure 12 Influenza deaths in Dublin in week ending 2 November 1918. (Source: Statistics derived from the weekly report of the registrar-general for 2 November 1918.)

Workhouses and influenza

Statistics on weekly workhouse deaths in the Dublin registration area confirm that deaths in workhouses increased substantially during the second and third waves of the epidemic. The LGB's annual report for the year ending March 1919, which includes most of the epidemic period, ascribed the elevated numbers of deaths in the workhouses during the year to influenza. Some 12,115 died in the workhouses in the year April 1918 – March 1919, an increase of 3,329 on the previous year. Most of the increase the LGB attributed to the influenza epidemics; deaths certified to 'influenza and pneumonia' increased by 2,551, and 'heart disease' by 527 on the previous year; the increase in deaths ascribed to heart disease suggests that certifying doctors considered the immediate cause of death to be heart disease, which may have been a sequela of influenza.[35] In the year to March 1920, 8,580 died in the workhouses, which was a decrease of 3,535 on the previous year.[36]

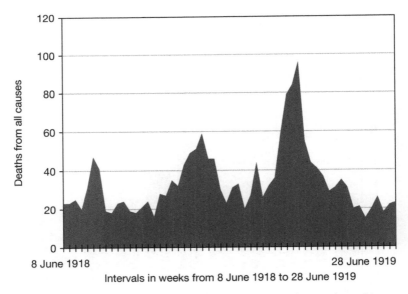

Figure 13 Deaths in workhouses in the Dublin area during the influenza epidemic.
(Source: weekly reports of the registrar general, 1918–19.)

Local Government Board statistics

The report mentioned that, because of the epidemic, the doctors of the Poor Law medical service made 100,000 extra visits to patients in their own homes compared to the previous year. This figure ought to be taken as a rough estimate, for several reasons. Thomas Hennessy has noted the difficulties that doctors had in actually documenting the numbers using the medical service. On average, the doctors attended 610,322 new cases each year, of which about one third were seen in the patients' own homes. He contended that even though that number sounded surprisingly high, it did not represent half of those who actually attended, particularly of patients who came to the dispensaries:

> The medical attendance on poor law patients is never registered unless they present tickets. Poor law patients, for different reasons, have an objection to providing tickets. Presentation of tickets to the dispensary doctor means no money to him; directly or indirectly. They only mean to him a huge amount of clerical work for which he has neither the time nor the inclination. The result is that he is agreeably pleased to be spared the trouble of registering them. His pleasure and satisfaction come in time to be appreciated and shared by the more observant of his patients, and thus it comes about that as many as half the cases attended by the dispensary doctors are not registered and are not included in the statistics given by the local government board.[37]

The Board itself admitted that influenza case figures were under-recorded, as it appeared that correct records had not been kept by some temporary medical officers during the influenza epidemic. From contemporary accounts during the epidemic, it would seem that each visit or ticket might cover several different people in the same household. With doctors such as Dr Rafferty working possibly eighteen-hour days, and visiting patients at all hours, it seems highly probable that they could not keep up with the paperwork, or would consider it a time-wasting exercise when they could be treating patients instead. The real number of new cases of influenza in the year ending March 1919 could therefore be much larger than the number of visits reported to the LGB.

Table 1 shows the impact that the pandemic made on the Poor Law dispensary service, as Poor Law MOHs made 100,000

Table 1 New cases attended by Poor Law medical officers of health in 1918–19.

New cases during year	Year ending March 1918	Year ending 31 March 1919	Year ending 31 March 1920
At dispensaries	428,015	424,182	396,467
In patients' homes	137,658	238,386	144,130
Total no. of new cases	565,673	662,568	540,597

Statistics taken from the annual reports of the Local Government Board for 1919 and 1920.

more house calls in the year to 31 March 1919 which contains all but one month of the three waves of the disease, than in the previous year.

Other statistical data relating to the influenza epidemic gleaned from the annual reports of the LGB includes a substantial increase in the cost of medicines to £31,545 in the year to March 1919, up from £26,253 in the previous year. Pay to temporary medical officers in the year to March 1919 was £27,247, increased from £17,624 on the previous year.[38] This figure represents a 55 per cent increase in the annual cost of temporary medical doctors, and is accounted for by the employment of replacement doctors during the influenza epidemic.

Limitation of the available data

The statistics compiled by the GRO have limitations. They do not represent the full picture of mortality from influenza, as influenza was sometimes misdiagnosed as other disease, and also because it seems possible that not all deaths were reported during this extremely busy period for doctors. This happened particularly in the early stages of the epidemic before doctors had realised what was happening; it also happened because the death classification system only permitted one cause of death, and reducing death to a single cause was not always that simple, particularly if a victim had a pre-existing condition like heart disease. A death from pneumonia or heart disease following influenza might be recorded in the statistics as a death from pneumonia or heart disease, even if the attending doctor had filled out the death certificate, as often happened, as 'pneumonia following influenza', 'influenzal pneumonia' or 'heart disease following influenza'. An early report comparing influenza and pneumonia mortality in 1918 in Dublin, New York, London and Paris found that the Dublin figures showed a relatively smaller proportion of deaths attributed to influenza and a relatively higher proportion of deaths attributed to pneumonia when compared to the London and Paris figures.[39] Many deaths were never recorded during the pandemic, the LGB admitted in an annual report, as doctors were too busy to do the paperwork.[40] Much of the more detailed information for influenza-specific deaths is only available for the larger cities, Dublin and Belfast, preventing, for example, an age-related examination of influenza deaths in smaller towns, unions or rural areas. The RG's office collated data on influenza and published the mortality tables contain a listing for influenza, but detailed data on influenza, for example weekly mortality and deaths by age, were only published for the Dublin registration area, meaning that it is not possible, for example, to chart the wave pattern of the influenza pandemic outside the capital city, or on a national basis. Even in Dublin, area-specific data on influenza was not published.

The Irish data on influenza permits only a limited level of analysis compared to, for example, data collected in England and Wales on the epidemic. George Newman's special report on influenza for the LGB of England and Wales contains such detailed information as to whether or not infants who died from influenza were being breast-fed. A survey of infants born to mothers suffering from influenza in London found that only 30 per cent of breast fed babies contracted the disease, whereas the attack rate in artificially fed infants was 54 per cent.[41] Newman's report also included a house to house survey on influenza in Leicester conducted by the Leicester MOH, Dr Arnold, who collated data on the numbers of rooms in the house, the number of residents with their sex, age and occupation, the dates on which residents had caught influenza, and details of their medical care during the attack. The LGB for Ireland did not issue a separate report on the influenza epidemic.[42]

Statisticians and historians using the methods of their disciplines to document the statistical incidence of pandemic influenza and other epidemic disease have tended to focus on the dead rather than on the difficulties that their loss caused their families. Accounts of Irish families whose circumstances were drastically altered by the loss of a parent to influenza are commonplace. Catherine Moran Heatley (aged twenty-four) died from 'influenzal pneumonia' in November 1918 in her parents' house in Nicholas Street, in Dublin's Liberties, with her three young sons at her bedside. She had been widowed when her husband Charles, a lance corporal with the Royal Dublin Fusiliers, was killed on 1 July 1916 at the Battle of the Somme. Their deaths left three young boys orphaned. James Delaney, a DMP constable stationed at Lad Lane died from 'pneumonia following influenza' in January 1919. His wife was forced by economic circumstance to work; she opened a business and their two children, Denis and Beck, were fostered for a time to grandparents living in the midlands. Tommy Christian's family unit was also broken up as a result of his mother's death from a sequela of influenza.[43] While accounts like these are not difficult to find in an Irish context, the available data is not sophisticated enough to easily count how many children were orphaned as a result of the pandemic. In contrast, Swedish statistics have enabled Elisabeth Engberg – an influenza researcher at the University of Umeå in Sweden – to map the social and kinship networks of influenza victims in Arjeplog, a rural parish in north central Sweden, in a fourth Swedish wave in 1920. She was able to survey living flu victims who had to cope with loss, changed social circumstances and sometimes extreme poverty in the aftermath of the pandemic. Engberg established that many of the dead were young parents, that 77 per cent of the surviving children were orphaned, and that only two of the twelve women widowed by influenza and one of the eight men widowed were in a position to hold their households together after their spouse died. Many families lost one parent; some lost both. In the case of widowers, remarriage usually offered the only chance to keep their families. In some cases, grown children refused to take care of elderly parents whose carers had been killed by the flu, with the result that they had to go into care. Only two widows were left in a comfortable financial position after the death of their spouses; both were the wives of independent farmers, with property and no debts.[44] It is not easy to find out from Irish statistics how many children were orphaned by Spanish influenza. How many family units were broken up as a result? How many had severely altered economic circumstances as a result of the death of the family breadwinner? These are unanswerable but interesting questions; oral histories of some families point to their individual traumas in Chapter 7.

Despite their limitations, the official statistics provide a further opportunity (adding to reasons cited earlier and later in this book) to query why the influenza epidemic was not considered worthy of attention by Irish historians in the past. At the most conservative estimate, just over 20,000 Irish people died in the influenza epidemic. The four cholera epidemics of the nineteenth century are familiar to the public and the historian alike, and feature on school syllabi. The cholera epidemic of 1832–35 killed an estimated 25,000 people in Ireland, while the epidemic associated with the Great Famine killed perhaps as many as 35,000. The other two cholera epidemics in Ireland, those of 1853–54 and 1866–67 had lower mortality.[45] Cholera killed 19,000 Irish people in 1832 alone, the year with the highest death toll in the 1832–35 epidemic, a total on a par with the 20,051 official deaths from influenza in 1918–19, given that most of these deaths took place within an eleven-month period from May or June 1918 to the end of April 1919.[46] Greta Jones has told that the tuberculosis epidemic, the leading cause of death in the nineteenth century and at the beginning of the twentieth century, attracted far less attention than the more dramatic epidemics of cholera, typhus and smallpox. She has suggested that part of the reason may be that these epidemics came and went in a dramatic fashion, and were often accompanied by social and economic crises.[47] The influenza epidemic was also a dramatic disease event, creating fear and paralysing communities as it passed through. The death statistics, flawed as they are, prove that it extracted a reasonably large, if not enormous, toll. Mortality estimates suggest that at least one in five people in Ireland caught the disease, placing the Irish experience of Spanish influenza on a par with conservative estimates of the international morbidity and mortality from the disease. This was the largest acute epidemic disease in Ireland in the twentieth century, meriting a place in history on the basis of statistical evidence alone. And yet, while the death statistics for the nineteenth-century cholera epidemics trip off the tongue of the secondary school history student, and are freely available in history textbooks, death statistics for this more recent disease event are not well known.

Notes

1 Roy Porter, *The Greatest Benefit to Mankind* (London: Fontana Press, 1999), pp. 407–8, 484–5.

2 Ibid., pp. 407–8.

3 Peter Froggatt, 'Sir William Wilde, 1815–1876: A Centenary Appreciation Wilde's Place in Medicine', Proceedings of the Royal Irish Academy. Section C: Archaeology, Celtic Studies, History, Linguistics, Literature Vol. 77 (1977), pp. 261–78. Wilde's expertise spanned his training in ophthalmic and aural surgery, and his interests in medicine, health, statistics, folklore, archaeology, history, topography and ethnology. Froggatt notes that Wilde was not, as some authorities suggest, assistant commissioner of the 1841 census. This is confirmed by James McGeachie, 'Wilde, Sir William Robert Wills (1815–1876)', *Oxford Dictionary of National Biography*, Oxford University Press, 2004, (www.oxforddnb.com/view/article/29403, accessed 27 July 2016).

4 World Health Organization website. From www.who.int/classifications/icd/en/HistoryOfICD.pdf, 9 June 2005.

5 B. Benjamin, *Elements of Vital Statistics* (London: Allen and Unwin, 1959), pp. 88–9.

6 Leo van Bergen, *Before my Helpless Sight* (Farnham: Ashgate, 2009), pp. 160–1. H.L. Dunn 'The evaluation of the effect upon mortality statistics of the selection of the primary cause of death', *Journal of the American Statistical Association*, xxxi, no. 193 (March, 1936), pp. 113–23.

7 E. Roesle, 'Classification of Causes of Deaths and Death Registration: Principle and Objects of the Classification of the Causes of Death', *Journal of the American Statistical Association*, xxi, no. 154 (June, 1926), pp. 195–205.

8 Charles Cameron, *Autobiography of Sir Charles Cameron* (Dublin: Hodges Figgis, 1921), pp. 140–2.

9 *Fifty-sixth annual report of the registrar-general for Ireland for 1919 (Births, Deaths, and Marriages)* (1920), xi, cmd 997.

10 *The Dublin Journal of Medical Science*, cxlv (1918), pp. 370–1.

11 Abdel R. Omran, 'The epidemiologic transition: a theory of the epidemiology of population change', *The Milbank Quarterly*, vol. 83, no. 4 (2005), pp. 731–57.

12 W.J. Thompson, 'Mortality from influenza in Ireland', *Journal of the Statistical and Social Inquiry Society of Ireland*, xiv, no. 1 (1919/20), pp. 1–14. W.J. Thompson, 'Mortality from influenza in Ireland', *Dublin Journal of Medical Science*, 4th series (1920), pp. 174–86.

13 *Fifty-fifth annual report of registrar-general for Ireland for 1918 (Births, Deaths, and Marriages)* (1919), x, cmd 450.

14 *Fifty-sixth annual report of registrar-general for Ireland for 1919.*

15 Edwin Oakes Jordan, *Epidemic Influenza: a Survey* (Chicago, IL: American Medical Association, 1927), p. 217.

16 Johnson, *Britain and the 1918–19 Influenza Pandemic*, p. 80.

17 *Fifty-sixth annual report of the registrar-general for Ireland.*

18 *Fifty-seventh annual report of registrar-general for Ireland for 1920 (Births, Deaths, and Marriages)* (1921), ix, cmd 1532. J.K. Taubenberger and D.M. Morens, '1918 influenza: the mother of all pandemics', *Emerging Infectious Diseases*, xii, no. 1 (January 2006), pp. 15–22.

19 The avian influenza or H5N1 epidemic of the twenty-first century continues, by stark contrast, to kill at least 50 per cent of its victims, and pneumonic plague would be expected to kill half its victims without medical care.

20 See, e.g., Elisabeth Engberg's work on the fourth wave in rural northern Sweden. Elisabeth Engberg, 'The invisible influenza: community response to pandemic influenza in rural northern Sweden 1918–20', *Vária Historia*, xlii, no. 25 (2009), pp. 429–56.

21 See Guy Beiner, Patricia Marsh and Ida Milne, 'Greatest killer of the twentieth century: the great flu in 1918–19, *History Ireland* (March–April 2009), pp. 40–3.

22 See Chapter 2.

23 Personal communication with Frank Taaffe, Dublin, 5 March 2011.

24 The Percy French song satirises the inefficiency of the West Clare Railway.

25 For a further discussion of the navies and influenza in Ireland, see Chapters 1, 4, 6 and 7.

26 See Jeffery Taubenberger, 'Genetic characterisation of the 1918 'Spanish' influenza virus', in Howard Phillips and David Killingray, eds, *The Spanish Influenza Pandemic of 1918–1919* (Abingdon: Routledge, 2003).

27 Centers for Disease Control and Prevention: 'Pregnant women & influenza (Flu)' www.cdc.gov/flu/protect/vaccine/pregnant.htm (accessed 16 January 2017).

28 Niall Johnson, 'Influenza in Britain in 1918–19', in Howard Phillips and David Killingray, eds, *The Spanish Influenza Pandemic of 1918–1919* (Abingdon: Routledge, 2003), p. 141.

29 *Fifty-fifth annual report of the registrar-general for Ireland. Fifty-sixth annual report of the registrar-general for Ireland.*

30 *Weekly returns of births and deaths for the Dublin registration area and in eighteen of the principal urban districts by the registrar-general for Ireland, 1918–1920.*

31 Svenn-Erik Mamelund, 'A socially neutral disease? Individual social class, household wealth and mortality from Spanish influenza in two

socially contrasting parishes in Kristiania 1918–19', in *Social Science & Medicine*, lxii, no. 4 (2006), pp. 923–40.

32 'Petty' from the French 'petit' meaning small or lower middle-class shopkeepers.

33 *Quarterly summary of the weekly returns of births and deaths in the Dublin registration area (October–December 1918).*

34 *Weekly return of births and deaths for the Dublin registration area and in eighteen of the principal urban districts for the week ending 2 November 1918.*

35 *Forty-seventh annual report of the Local Government Board for Ireland for the year ended 31 March 1919* (1920), xxi, cmd 578.

36 *Forty-eight annual report of the Local Government Board* (for England and Wales), *1918–1919* (1920), xxiv, cmd 413.

37 *Medical Press*, 'Medical reform for Ireland', 12 February 1919.

38 *Forty-seventh annual report of the Local Government Board for Ireland.*

39 W.H. Frost and Edgar Sydenstricker, 'Epidemic influenza in foreign countries', *Public Health Reports (1896–1970)*, xxxiv, no. 25 (20 June, 1919), pp. 1361–76.

40 During the course of this work, it was found that many influenza victims' deaths had not been recorded; death certification was more likely if the victim was male. See Chapter 4.

41 *Forty-eighth annual report of the Local Government Board (for England and Wales), 1918–1919, supplement containing the report of the Medical Department for 1918–19* (1919), cmd 462.

42 Ibid.

43 See Chapter 6.

44 Elisabeth Engberg, 'Caring for the fatherless: epidemic influenza and family dissolution in Sweden, 1920', paper presented to the ESSHC conference, Ghent, April 2010; and personal communications.

45 S.J. Connolly, ed., *The Oxford Companion to Irish History* (Oxford: Oxford University Press, 1998), p. 87.

46 Gerard O'Brien, 'State intervention and medical relief of the poor', in Greta Jones and Elizabeth Malcolm, eds, *Medicine, Disease and the State in Ireland, 1650–1940* (Cork: Cork University Press, 1998), pp. 195–207.

47 Jones, 'The campaign against tuberculosis in Ireland, 1899–1914', pp. 158–76.

4

'Managing' the crisis

How medical care was organised and managed in early twentieth-century Ireland? How did patients access the system? What role did the Government play in the pandemic, through its local agents bearing responsibility for overseeing public health and sanitation, the Local Government Board for Ireland?

This chapter argues that the influenza epidemic, by placing pressure on the medical system and its institutions, highlighted pre-existing tensions between the LGB and the BOGs as local administrators of the Poor Law dispensary system, and problems over the terms and conditions of employment of the Poor Law MOHs. It shows that the LGB, like the LGB for England and Wales, was perceived by the press and many of the BOGs to take a back seat in the management of the disease, rather than devising a central plan. This left the management to the local agents of the Poor Law dispensary service (i.e. the BOGs), to individual hospitals and local authorities, and to schemes set up by local charitable organisations and communities. In some part, these were appropriate delegations, as responses to epidemics need to be local in nature, and local authorities had statutory obligations in relation to sanitation and notifiable diseases. The local authorities' medical officers of health – in some areas – relished the challenge, and became proactive in presenting suggestions to the public and to businesses on how to handle it. Charles Cameron, the veteran MOH for Dublin Corporation became the reporters' favourite source for quotes and advice. In other areas, pioneering doctors, journalists and charitable societies devised localised strategies for nursing and feeding the ill.

The official handling of the crisis

As the world war lumbered towards an end, sharp rises in the price of food and scarcity of fuel reduced people's buying power and inflicted real hardship on those on lower incomes. The alarming deterioration in social conditions led to industrial unrest as trade unions organised a movement to negotiate better pay in 1918 to enable workers to afford the higher costs of living.[1] The war, which was brought closer by returning soldiers and U-boat activity in the Irish Sea, also increased dangers to, and fears about dangers to, public health. Both in Great Britain and in Ireland there was an awareness that infectious diseases, such as smallpox, typhus and dysentery, could spread from regions devastated by the war. The increased costs of food staples like bread, milk and eggs, allied with the scarcity of coal, led to an apprehension that the resistance of, in particular, the urban poor, to disease would be weakened, something often discussed in the newspapers. In response, efforts were made by the Dublin Castle administration and by local authorities to control the price of essential commodities and to provide coal for the most vulnerable in order to increase the physical defences of the urban poor to disease. The war also led to a retrenchment on spending on services not directly related to the war effort; services that did relate directly to the war effort also impinged on the medical care of the civilian population, including an embargo on filling medical posts in the Poor Law dispensary service, and the treatment of war wounded and the ill in the civilian hospitals.[2] Even before the war, the professional medical organisations had been battling to improve the pay and pension terms and conditions of Poor Law doctors, while an Irish derogation from the 1911 National Insurance Act meant that, unlike their counterparts in England and Wales, insured workers did not have their medical care covered, placing an added load on the Poor Law medical system.[3] The additional pressures provided by such a large scale influenza epidemic exacerbated these festering problems. These factors, and the tense political situation, formed the backdrop to the Irish influenza crisis.

The patient in the medical system

An influenza epidemic begins with the individual sufferer. To look at how the healthcare system worked, it is expedient to look at how the patient fitted into that system. During the 1918–19 epidemic, a two-tier medical system was in operation. Which tier the patient was treated under depended on their economic situation, rather than the degree of illness. Those who could afford it called on the family doctor to attend, usually a person who was part of the circle of family acquaintances. If the doctor deemed it necessary, they might have been able to secure the services of a private nurse to care for them. Hospital care was not usually an option for the affluent unless they became extremely ill, and even then, there was a possibility that the care would be in a private nursing home attached to a voluntary hospital rather than on a public ward.[4] Good nursing, most authorities have agreed then and since, was the best path to recovery, and in this pre-antibiotic era, there was not much that medicine could do except alleviate the symptoms, given that for many the killer was pneumonia.[5] For the poor – and this category tended to be a loose description – there was the Poor Law medical dispensary system. As Thomas Hennessy, Irish medical secretary of the British Medical Association, explained to members of the Royal Academy of Medicine in Ireland in an address on medical reform for Ireland, in practice rather than in theory, this system covered between 50 and 70 per cent of the Irish population.[6] The medical benefits of the 1911 National Insurance Act did not apply in Ireland; insured workers could receive illness benefit – as Peter Martin notes a cash payment – their medical treatment was not covered in the same way as their counterparts under the system in England and Wales.[7] So unlike the position in England and Wales, most workers in Ireland, even if they subscribed to the national insurance schemes, had to receive their medical treatment under the Poor Law scheme, which, in turn, meant that general practitioners were deprived of more paying patients.

To receive treatment under the Poor Law, there was a ticketing system: black for presentation and treatment at a Poor Law dispensary; and red for attendance by a MOH employed by the local BOGs at the patient's home. If the patient required more care and treatment than the doctor or family and neighbours could provide, they were removed to hospital. In country areas, this was a cumbersome journey, often of many miles on rough roads in horse-drawn or motor ambulances. Admission to hospital was not a simple process either.[8] There were differing criteria for admission to hospitals, which varied according to institution. In the county infirmaries, members of the committees of management gave orders for the admission of patients. Admission to Poor Law union infirmaries and fever hospitals was indirect. The patient was first supposed to be admitted to the workhouse on the authority of the relieving officer, or in an emergency, on the authority of the master. The medical officer of the workhouse then had to decide whether the person so admitted was to be sent to the infirmary, to the fever hospital, or to the body of the house. This system may explain the reluctance of people ill with flu to receive medical attention in the workhouse infirmary, as there was a persistent fear that they might end up in the workhouse as inmates rather than patients. At the height of the epidemic, workhouse infirmaries were under such pressure that some had to use other parts of the workhouse to care for the ill.[9] Medical practitioners had no power to give orders for the admission of a patient to any rate-aided hospital, unless they held a post as dispensary medical officer, and then only to the few fever hospitals under the control of the sanitary authorities. The voluntary hospitals run by charitable organisations also had diverse admission criteria.[10] The Adelaide, for example, admitted only Protestant patients (see Chapter 6 for a further discussion of the impact of the pandemic on hospitals).

The epidemic and Poor Law medical system

The vast majority of Spanish influenza sufferers did not go to hospital. Some of the estimated one fifth of the population who showed symptoms had relatively mild attacks, and hence the burden of care for the rest fell on the private practitioners and the practitioners in the employ of the BOGs who administrated the Poor Law medical dispensary system at a local level, and on whoever was available to nurse them.[11] Only the more severe cases, which usually meant those with respiratory or pneumonic complications, were removed to hospital, if space permitted. Newspaper reports document the extra pressures that the huge numbers of influenza patients placed on the BOGs and their employees. The account referred to in Chapter 2, which was related by Dr Rafferty of Rathdown Union and published in the *Wicklow People* on 19 October 1918, appears to be typical of the experience of the MOHs during the epidemic. Dispensary doctors worked around the clock to care for their patients. They could have, Thomas Hennessy suggested, 4,000 or 5,000 people solely dependent on them for medical care in a dispensary district covering an area of 144 square miles.[12]

Close contact with vast numbers of ill patients, coupled with the long hours they worked, made them more vulnerable to catching the disease themselves. Then the burden fell on the BOGs through the relieving officers to find temporary replacements, and when the replacements fell ill, replacements in turn for them. All this was rendered more difficult by a shortage of staff due to doctors falling prey to the disease, by demands for higher locum fees from a medical profession who suddenly found their bargaining power increased, and by the reluctance of the LGB, as reported by several BOGs, to sanction the payment of those higher fees. To add to the crisis, many doctors were elderly, and forced by poor pension arrangements to continue working, and this was compounded by the embargo in force since 1915 on doctors young enough for army service being appointed to permanent posts in the dispensary service; many hospital and dispensary doctors were on leave from their posts to serve in the armed forces. Some of these elderly doctors paid a heavy price for attending diligently to their duties during the epidemic.

Reports from the Carlow *Nationalist* on 9 November 1918 about the relieving officers' difficulties in finding doctors to cover the work of ill Union medical officers are typical of the experience all over Ireland during the peak weeks of the epidemic. At the beginning of the second week in November, the epidemic had spread to Tullow and Baltinglass. Carlow dispensary's Dr Doyle was ill with flu, and the relieving officer, Mr Brennan, had appointed Dr Ryan in his place for a week at the rate the guardians had recently fixed for *locum tenens*, five guineas per week. Dr MacCarthy of Tullow Hospital was also ill, and relieving officer Mr Fanning had appointed Dr Kidd to do duty at the hospital at £3 weekly. Dr Dundon had refused to do further duty except at ten guineas per week, prepaid.[13] Dr Fisher had been appointed to do duty at Bagnalstown hospital, in place of the ill Dr Farrell. After three days, Fisher himself fell ill, and the relieving officer Mr Kelly had to search for another, appointing Dr MacDonald for one day, and then Dr Myers from Dublin for four days at £2 10s per day. Kelly tried to recruit other doctors, who asked for £3 per day plus expenses. He eventually appointed Dr Banley at a fee of four guineas per week. Doctors employed as locums by the Dublin Union were receiving six guineas a week in November 1918, a rise of a guinea on the previous month.[14] In Naas Union, some doctors were receiving seven guineas per week by November 1918.

The minutes of the Naas guardians' meetings placed on record the guardians' great appreciation of the diligent work done by not only the union doctors and nurses, but also by the relieving officers and the guardians themselves during the epidemic. Their own families were often influenza victims. At a meeting on 10 December, they offered sympathy to the vice-chairman, Mr Gogarty, who had a general merchant and hardware business on the Main Street, on the death of his daughter (a milliner in Canada), brother and nephew from the disease; his son had died from influenza a few weeks earlier; and another daughter died in January 1919 from influenza as well. All but one of these fatalities, a nun living in Belgium, worked in retail.[15] Naas was a black spot for influenza, with particular local factors worsening the situation. A letter to the guardians from Dr M.R. Morrissey illustrates the extreme calls on the service during the peak weeks of the epidemic:

> When I came to Naas on Sunday 13th ultimo (October) I heard Dr Murphy was sick and called to see him when he told me he had between 300 and 400 cases of influenza in the town. Shortly afterwards, Mr Carroll, relieving officer, asked me to take up duty in Naas. I agreed to do so for some days at three guineas a day ... I found matters even still worse than I thought, as I was kept going day and night with fresh cases every hour. This continued during the week. There were 50 or 60 red tickets every day, and each ticket represented four to ten persons. By 20 October there were about a thousand cases in the town. As the epidemic began to spread to the country and these cases took up so much of my time, I found that I could not do this alone, and I requested you and Mr Carroll, relieving officer, to provide me with another doctor and some nurses. I required the latter to look after the pneumonia cases of which a good number suffered at this period. In many houses every member was confined to bed and no person to look after them. Here again the nurses were necessary. Dr Fitzpatrick took up duty and looked after most of the patients on the south side of the town whilst I did the north side and most of the country calls. I roughly estimate that by 26 October there were 1,420 in Naas and immediate districts ... There is certainly a word of praise due to Nurse Mooney for the able work she did in the early part of the epidemic before she got assistance. Her attention and care saved many pneumonic cases.[16]

Workhouse infirmaries quickly filled up during the peak weeks of the epidemic in the Leinster area. In Dublin Union workhouse, the master, on the recommendations of the infirmary doctor, vacated four wards in the male hospital occupied by the 'feeble infirm and ulcer cases', moving them to the workhouse proper, to cater for influenza patients at the end of October 1918. The master took on extra nursing staff and appointed a man to ensure the swift removal of the bodies of patients who died during the night. The increased number of admissions also placed an added demand on the workhouse's cab and ambulance service, and extra staff had to be taken on to cater for that demand. The ambulance was, when necessary, loaned out to bring flu victims to hospitals.[17] In the eastern half of the province, workhouse infirmaries (sometimes known as 'Union hospitals' or 'the Union') and fever hospitals were reported to be full during the peak weeks of the epidemic in the autumn and winter of 1918 and the spring of 1919; the situation was particularly grim in Wexford town and New Ross, Kilkenny city, Athy, Naas and Dundalk at the end of October and in November. Extra nursing staff had to be taken on, particularly for the night shifts. Keeping the ill warm in dispensaries and infirmaries also required extra supplies of coal and someone to stoke the fires. There were constant complaints about coal running out in workhouses during the epidemic. Keeping medicines in stock was also a difficulty, because of heavy demand for medicines used to treat influenza and because the ordering system was so cumbersome that it usually took several weeks for supplies to arrive. Some BOGs ordered pharmaceutical supplies by telephone and got them delivered by train at the request of dispensary doctors. In the Dublin Union, some dispensary doctors hired pharmacists or compounders to take over the task of making up medicines, which freed them up to see patients.[18]

Unnecessary hardships were sometimes caused by minor logistical issues. Two families from Newtownbarry (Bunclody) were refused admission to Enniscorthy fever hospital because the hospital doctor considered it full. The union clerk pointed out there were only twenty-one patients in the hospital which was supposed to accommodate sixty-seven. As all the beds were occupied, he suggested moving more from the workhouse into the fever hospital.

Newspaper reports, even from those newspapers considered to be pro-establishment, documented the persistent grumbles and negative feelings of many of the BOGs and the dispensary staffs towards the

LGB, which was perceived to be out of touch with the needs of the day. A circular issued by the LGB at the height of the epidemic, as its agents struggled to provide for the medical needs of thousands of influenza sufferers in their unions, serves to illustrate that remoteness. Circulated in November 1918, it urged strict economy with coal, recommending people have fewer hot meals, less frequent hot baths and smaller fires. The situation was almost farcical given that the LGB's own recommendations for influenza prevention included good nourishment and keeping patients warm and clean, and contemporary influenza treatments made strong demands on hot water and required patients to be kept adequately heated and hydrated. The outrage caused by the circular caused was covered in many newspapers.[19]

Other incidences of the board's normal exacting book-keeping indicate its failure to appreciate the scale and suffering of the epidemic and the pressures lower down their medical system, and the need to adapt to the situation, in the exceptional circumstances of the pandemic. The LGB wrote to some BOGs complaining that they had paid too much for whiskey during the epidemic. The Youghal board responded that they had been very lucky to get whiskey at any price. The LGB refused to sanction a gratuity of £75 each voted to three medical officers by the Enniscorthy Guardians for extra work performed during the epidemic; the board said that they saw no reason why doctors should receive extra payments because the volume of their work in a given period was above the average. The chairman of Enniscorthy Guardians, Mr H.A. Lett, considered the LGB's attitude 'most unfair', and a special meeting was convened to discuss the matter. The Rathdown Guardians, at their meeting on 19 February 1919, were outraged that the LGB 'refused to allow Dr Pim one shilling' for all the work he did as medical officer of the workhouse. Dr Pim had 325 additional patients; Mr Barrington Jellett said he wished to repeat in the strongest possible terms that the officials who declined to sanction this £20 bonus deliberately fixed at a low amount to preclude any possible objection from the LGB, had very little sense of their responsibilities to the poor of the Rathdown district, and that he considered the refusal to sanction the bonus a public scandal. A unanimous resolution was passed protesting at the action of the LGB and requesting a revision of their decision to reject Pim's bonus.

The LGB was arguably the public face of government in Ireland, with its members being better known than officials at Dublin Castle through their interaction with the local authorities and the BOGs who administered the Poor Law health system at local level. In the lead up to the influenza crisis, relations between the mainly nationalist BOGs and the LGB had been deteriorating.[20] As Sir Henry Robinson, the long-term vice-president and *de facto* head of the LGB, observed in his second memoir:

> The LGB, because of its drastic powers for regulating local expenditure by governing bodies, was naturally regarded by the patriotic local Guardians and Councillors as the statutory Saxon curse of the country and a department which could never appreciate the high spirited Irish contempt for the restriction of dirty little English Acts of Parliament.[21]

When the LGB failed to take a proactive stance on the developing health crisis in the summer and autumn of 1918, appearing out of touch with the situation, few were surprised. The issue became one more spark point between the government and its discontented local agents, the BOGs, who administered the Poor Law at local level.

The influenza and doctors: politics and pay

The LGB's dogmatic insistence on tight control of Poor Law doctors' fees during the influenza crisis became a major issue between them and the Poor Law BOGs. Just as the overwhelming scale of the influenza epidemic exposed flaws within the government system of public health and sanitation and exacerbated other ongoing disputes, the epidemic reignited a long-running dispute over the emoluments paid to the Poor Law's MOHs. Complaints from Irish dispensary doctors and their advocates about the size of their districts, their meagre salaries, and the categories of people for whom they were required to provide medical care were frequently recorded in the pages of the *British Medical Journal* in the fifty years before the epidemic; little had been done to meet these calls for reform.[22] Thomas Hennessy pointed out that between 50 and 70 per cent of the Irish population could claim free medical care; this meant more work for the doctors under the dispensary system, and less private practice work and therefore less private practice income. The Poor Law MOHs claimed to be badly paid, and had unsatisfactory pension and holiday rights. Proposals to resolve the situation by extending the medical benefits of the national insurance scheme to Ireland, recommended in 1913 by a departmental committee appointed by the Treasury, had never been implemented. Doctors of an age to serve in the military were banned by the LGB from appointment to Poor Law medical posts; this imposed pressures on the Poor Law medical system long before the influenza epidemic occurred.[23] Doctors were overworked and some had to work well into old age because they had no pension. They had to bargain individually to get increases in expenses for fuel and transport costs. At the time of the influenza epidemic, transport costs had, like most other commodities towards the end of the war, increased substantially, and doctors were obliged to use transport more than ever to tend to the vast numbers of influenza ill. Many claimed to be out of pocket as a result, their Poor Law expenses inadequate to cover their expenditure. The flu gave doctors a scarcity value: as many posts had to be filled with locums on a temporary basis when doctors became ill or died, a higher value was placed on their services. Influenza, by placing further pressure on that already overtaxed system, presented the Poor Law doctors with more bargaining power for their demands for increased salaries.

The two doctors' associations used the opportunity to politicise their goals. *The Irish Supplement to the Medical Press*, the official organ of the Irish Medical Association, urged its members to use the December 1918 general election to canvass candidates about medical reforms, and demand that they pledge support for compulsory superannuation for the Poor Law MOHs.[24] In an article noting that the fees for *locum tenens* had improved, and that the movement for increased salaries for the Poor Law service was progressing steadily, they encouraged doctors to keep applying political pressure to secure fair rates for salaries. The Irish Medical Association feared that when army was demobilised army doctors would be thrown onto the employment market, and, following the increase in numbers of doctors looking for work, that salaries would again be reduced to what they termed 'starvation' rates. In October 1918, the army alone was employing more than 13,150 medical doctors, compared to 3,800 before the war. The Irish branch of the British Medical Association had held a delegate meeting on 29 May 1918 to discuss the salaries and conditions of service of Poor Law MOHs. The meeting also passed a resolution in favour of extending medical benefits of the national insurance scheme to Ireland on conditions acceptable to the profession. Following the meeting, the association petitioned all the BOGs in Ireland for increased salaries for their Poor Law MOHs. Many of the boards readily admitted the inadequacy of the salaries of their Poor Law MOHs, and, in some instances, granted fairly substantial increases in the case of doctors with long service. However, the LGB refused to sanction maximal salaries of £250 per annum on the ground of their being excessive. A deputation of Poor Law MOHs and the Irish Medical Secretary met the Board to give a detailed account of the financial difficulties of Poor Law MOHs in discharging their duties efficiently owing to their inadequate salaries, and pointed out that, as the result of the war, these difficulties had become intolerable, given the enormous increases in the cost of living and travelling. Soon after the meeting, the LGB contacted the BOGs concerned and informed them that it had decided to sanction maximum salaries of £250 per annum in the case of medical officers who had completed fifteen years of service and upwards.[25] Over 100 BOGs granted increases to their medical officers during the year to the end of March 1919, with eighty boards revising and augmenting scales of pay during the same year. The process continued during the following year, and by the end of March 1920, 150 of the 154 BOGs had granted their doctors some salary increase, graded scales or bulk sums. The LGB admitted that some of these increases were not commensurate with the needs of the times and the merits of the claims. Four BOGs refused time after time to make any increase.[26]

The epidemic and local authority and community initiatives

Local authorities were vested, under the Public Health Acts, with powers to administer the sanitary acts and regulations and also with functions relating to the provision of hospital facilities. As the bodies responsible for sanitation, they had specific duties during the pandemic. In Dublin and in other towns, many local authorities introduced the practice of disinfecting streets on a daily basis during the peak weeks of the second and third waves.[27] A particularly thorough programme of disinfection was considered to be a factor in Enniscorthy not suffering so badly in the initial stages of the second wave compared to its neighbouring towns.

In the absence of visible public leadership during the influenza epidemic from Dublin Castle or the LGB, key figures in local politics and sanitation took the initiative. Chief among these were Dublin Corporation's MOH, Sir Charles Cameron, and the city's Lord Mayor, Laurence O'Neill. Cameron, eighty-eight years old, had worked to improve the health of Dubliners for half a century, and was constantly sought out by journalists looking for influenza advice to give to their readers. His contributions were clear, cautious and practical. He advised that most of the complications of influenza were caused by people getting out of bed before they were completely recovered.[28] Cameron's advice in a letter published in the *Evening Herald* on 10 October, was typical:

> Sir,
>
> Influenza of the epidemic form has reappeared in a few districts of the city and may spread to other districts. It is very desirable that children should not be sent to school for the present.
>
> Those who feel unwell, possibly from the beginning of an attack should at once send for their physician and go to bed. Those recovering from the malady should not leave the house until advised by their physician.[29]

Many business premises were voluntarily disinfected every day during the pandemic, on the advice of Sir Charles Cameron. At his suggestion, the cinema houses 'responded favourably' to requests not to admit children of school age; they also closed for half an hour between shows to allow for the ventilation of the premises, and used approved disinfecting preparations freely. The Corporation's Public Health Department officials inspected city venues to check whether they were taking the proper precautions to curtail the dissemination of the disease in crowded situations. Again on Cameron's advice, the technical schools were closed and posters were published, giving precautionary advice. As the *Irish Times* remarked: 'Disinfection and purification are the watchwords just now with housekeepers and managers of all sorts of business and general establishments.'

O'Neill, whose influence was such that the newspapers often only referred to him as 'the Lord Mayor' even when he was in Belfast, was a negotiator of some repute, and a highly respected politician. His initiative and ability to solve problems were put to good effect several times during the influenza crisis. In mid-October, he helped to settle a strike in ten businesses in the Dublin undertakers' trade that was causing delays in burials.[30] He also negotiated the conditional release of Sinn Féin activist and doctor Kathleen Lynn so that she could work with influenza victims, and was called in to negotiate between Sinn Féin prisoners and prison authorities in Belfast jail in a long-running dispute over how the DORA (Defence of the Realm Act) prisoners who were suffering from influenza should be treated.[31] O'Neill was a member of the Public Health Committee of Dublin Corporation, which kept a close eye on the progress of the disease and the latest reports from Sir Charles Cameron. The chairman of the committee, P.T. Daly, Cameron and his deputy, Dr Matthew Russell, visited Dublin hospitals on 23 October 1918 to assess the accommodation available for influenza patients. They found that many of the beds were occupied by soldiers, and decided to approach the military authorities to ask them to provide accommodation for military patients other than in the civilian hospitals. The military authorities agreed to stop sending soldiers to civilian hospitals with effect from 24 October.[32]

The Public Health Committee, perhaps seeking to redress rather convoluted advice issued by the LGB in a public memorandum in late October (see below), issued their own practical advice on methods of avoiding and treating influenza in November 1918:

1. Keep away from crowded assemblies.
2. Do not spit on the floor or tramcar or on the streets. Expectorated matter may be full of objectionable microbes. In sneezing keep a handkerchief on your face, keep a little pad of cotton containing eucalyptus and smell it often, especially when in contact with other people.
3. Allow plenty of air into your dwelling. Avoid crowded rooms.
4. Vermin and dirt convey contagion. The strictest cleanliness should be observed.
5. Do not over exert yourself or give way to panic.
6. If you feel a pain in the head, or feverish, go to bed, and send for a doctor.
7. In recovering from influenza only see the persons you are obliged to see, so as to avoid infecting others.[33]

The epidemic's third wave caused the highest death rates from all causes on record in Dublin, and this was against a background trend of rapidly declining death rates from infectious disease.[34] The corporation's Public Health Committee invited representatives of the city hospitals to a conference at the public health office to explore whether sufficient hospital accommodation could be provided for influenza-pneumonia cases. They were told that the hospitals were under financial pressure due to greatly increased costs, and that accommodation could not be provided unless the corporation undertook to pay a sum of five shillings per day for each patient. If the corporation would agree to do so, the hospital authorities would be able to provide the necessary beds, nursing assistance and medical care. In the circumstances the committee agreed to ask the council to accede to this request, and authorised the MOH to issue admission orders where necessary. The chairman of the Public Health Committee referred to this arrangement at a special meeting of the Dublin municipal council held on 25 February 1919, mentioning that the finance committee had already sanctioned a provision to cover the cost in the coming year.[35]

This council meeting, chaired by O'Neill, was called with the intent of making influenza-pneumonia a notifiable disease for six months under the Infectious Disease (Notification) Act, 1889, on the advice of Cameron and Dr Matthew Russell. Under the provisions of this act, the local authorities were required to supervise the notification of certain listed infectious diseases; they could also add other diseases as they considered it necessary. The issue of making influenza-pneumonia a notifiable disease was not as straightforward a decision as it appeared. Various contributors to the council discussion argued that such a move would place extra cost on the poor as there was a one-shilling notification fee, and that in cases where a household occupied one room, it would not be possible to isolate a patient and they would be obliged to go to hospital, thus presenting the possibility of a further economic imposition on the poor. There was also an issue with ambulances, as cases of 'contagious' disease could not be transported to hospital by the police or the fire brigade so the Public Health Committee would have to supply their own staff. The LGB's Dr Browne considered it highly desirable that the disease should be notifiable, as it gave public health officials increased powers to deal with the disease. Dr Browne, Dr Russell and Sir Charles Cameron said they had decided that it was not necessary to make influenza notifiable on its own.[36] Of the move, the outspoken Kathleen Lynn was to note, slightly inaccurately, in her diary: 'Influenza notifiable now, they were long about it.'[37] The meeting also approved a motion empowering the Public Health Committee to spend £1,000 to employ extra nurses and to provide extra nursing necessities during the epidemic.

Some proactive local authorities and BOGs, although lacking the resources that Dublin Corporation had to call on, issued advice on various public health issues to do with the epidemic. Athy Urban District Council ordered one of sanitary officers to disinfect, fumigate and limewash the houses of influenza victims, and remove the dung heaps in alleyways, which were believed to be contributing to the problem. Like many of the more proactive local authorities, the Athy UDC advised against the holding of wakes, and also advised that influenza victims should be placed in coffins and buried as quickly as possible.[38] Some local authorities in the smaller towns appealed, through the pages of local newspapers, for the 'good ladies of the town' and charitable organisations to assist in the cooking and delivering of hot food for the sick, usually with a positive response. Apart from the communal kitchens discussed in Chapter 2, local branches of St Vincent de Paul and the WNHA helped out in many areas. Some landlords provided food for their tenants and employees, and neighbours helped each other. Mrs Barton from Straffan House in north Kildare was driven around in her carriage, bringing food and soup to the ill. Lady Mayo from Palmerstown House visited houses with soup and milk puddings. Lady Mayo also donated food to the WNHA soup kitchen in Naas. In Rathvilly, Co. Carlow, the Rathdonnells of Lisnaveagh brought hot soup down to the villagers, as Nellie O'Toole related (see Chapter 7). In Tipperary, the Clonmel Borstal and the Red Cross fed the ill of the town until funds were raised locally for a community kitchen operation (see Chapter 6).

National insurance

National insurance offered some financial protection to workers who caught the disease, even though it did not pay for medical care (a deviation from the practice in the neighbouring island). This meant that at least insured workers had some meagre income to tide them over while out of work with influenza. In all, 746,000 workers were paying into national insurance schemes in Ireland in the half-year ending June 1918; 503,000 were male and 243,000 were female. The 1921 report of National Health Insurance Commission (Ireland), discussing the period November 1917 to 31 March 1920, mentioned an increase of the funds issued to approved societies for benefits and expenses of administration was 'doubtless accounted for in great measure by the successive epidemics of influenza which were general throughout the country in these years'. From 1 July 1918, fully insured (i.e. with 104 weeks' payment) male workers could claim a sickness benefit of ten shillings a week; the rate for similarly qualified female workers was seven shillings and six pence; men with a minimum of twenty-six weeks of contributions qualified for a sickness benefit of six shillings a week and women five shillings a week. All payments were subject to the meeting of certain conditions. Tables 2 and 3 show the net sickness benefits paid to workers who paid their insurance through approved societies for the years 1917–19, and the sickness benefits for the same period paid to individual deposit contributors, showing the average sum paid for each sickness claim. The numbers of deposit contributors were small relative to the other group; in the six months to June 1918, there were a total of 2,238 deposit contributors; this number dropped to 1,896 in the last six months of 1918. The acute rise in sickness benefit paid to men in 1919 may be in part accounted for by an increased membership of discharged soldiers, which impedes assessment of the impact of the influenza on disability payments.[39]

Table 2 Sickness benefits paid to approved societies for the years 1917–19.

Benefits/net	1917/£	1918/£	1919/£	Members in June 1918
Men	183,534	225,009	204,125	502,833
Women	91629	104,609	93,853	243,247
Total				746,080

From the report of the National Health Insurance Commission (Ireland) 1921.

Table 3 Sickness benefits paid to deposit contributors during the years 1917–19.

Year	Gender	Number of payments	Total	Average amounts per payment
1917	Men	677	£472 6s 8d	13s 11d
	Women	884	£557 15s 8d	12s 7d
1918	Men	764	£557 6s 7d	14s 7d
	Women	861	£545	12s 8d
1919	Men	947	£797 11s 4d	16s 10d
	Women	889	£561 4s 2d	12s 8d

From the report of the National Health Insurance Commission (Ireland) 1921.

The Government, transport and influenza

The disease entered Ireland through infected people coming by ship; the government played both direct and indirect roles in containing the spread of influenza by ship and rail. The exceptional number of soldiers coming to Ireland by ship and train, on leave, to convalesce or returning following demobilisation, has been suggested by Catriona Foley and Patricia Marsh as a significant factor in spreading the disease. On the one hand, this is an attractive proposition: after all, the Irish rail network was at its most extensive length ever in 1918; demobilisation involved mass movement of soldiers from areas where influenza was rampant, from the arenas of war and through Great Britain. There are precedents, for this happened in other countries. D. Ann Herring and Lisa Sattenspiel wrote of sick soldiers bringing the flu by train to Winnipeg in Manitoba on 30 September 1918; four days later soldiers and a railway worker were dead, and within a fortnight influenza was rampant in the city.[40]

The Irish position, however, is more nuanced that it would initially appear. The bulk of demobilisation to Ireland occurred after the influenza pandemic had passed. Further work needs to be done on demobilisation before we could make definitive assertions about its bearing on the spread of the disease. There is little evidence or even comment in the official statistics, contemporary newspapers or in the archives of the railways to indicate that rail travel was a major agent in the spread of the disease, whether among the military or the civilian populations.[41] Mass assemblies like anti-conscription rallies, sporting events and race meetings, the celebrations for the end of the war, funerals and the general election rallies and celebrations would seem far more effective as a means of spreading influenza than the narrow confines of a rail carriage, and in any case, special trains were often run exclusively for moving large groups of soldiers. A handful of returning soldiers infected with influenza may explain sporadic outbreaks in areas where Spanish influenza was not yet endemic, but there is as yet no compelling evidence for major regional outbreaks of influenza in Ireland owing to rail travel, by soldiers or civilians. Train journeys may have been the locus of infection from influenza for some civilians, including perhaps for John Ralph and Sam Williamson of Co. Wexford, as mentioned in Chapter 7; it would be difficult to avoid catching influenza when sharing a small train compartment for several hours with a sneezing and coughing sufferer. But it does not seem convincing as a major factor in the dissemination of the disease in the Ireland. For one thing, passenger railway services were greatly curtailed in 1918 because of the coal shortage. The reduction of coal imports into Ireland by 20 per cent announced in March 1918 forced the Great Southern and Western Railway (GSWR) to reduce drastically the number of passenger trains, curtailing scheduled services by 29 per cent from 22 April. Their passenger train mileage in 1918 was decreased by 643,745, or 18 per cent less than the previous year. The authorities considered it judicious, given the food shortages being experienced around the country, to preserve coal for trains carrying goods and livestock, 'as a war necessity of paramount importance'. Passenger travel on the railways was further discouraged by the Railways Passenger Fares Ireland Order 1918, which authorised an advance of 50 per cent in passenger fares from 1 June. While the GSWR continued to run special trains for the military, most of these were for military patrols rather than for soldiers on leave or returning from the war arena.[42] On the other hand, there is some evidence that the presence of naval vessels in Lough Swilly may have played a factor in Donegal experiencing high level of infection throughout the pandemic period, rather than in one or two waves. The other issue is that there was a lot of civilian traffic in ferries and other ships across the Irish Sea, which undoubtedly helped to spread the disease.

The War Office, aware of incidences of high morbidity and mortality from influenza on overcrowded American and New Zealand troop transport ships, and wary also of the possibility that returning soldiers could spread influenza and other infectious disease among the civilian populations in Britain to which they were returning, introduced measures to prevent or curtail the spread of influenza on board transports from September 1918. Soldiers who were due to sail home on leave were detained in camps for fourteen days before embarkation and were not allowed to embark if they were considered to be suffering from or incubating influenza or other infectious disease. All forms of transport on the North American (which would have included those passing around Ireland) and New Zealand routes were fitted with steam spray disinfection chambers; the space between hammocks and bunks was increased, and ill soldiers were detained in one section of the transport. When the period of demobilisation arrived, the War Office recognised that the risk of spreading flu from contacts on board ship increased, as the men went to their homes within one or two days of their arrival in Britain. It was arranged that a special medical examination should be made of all troops on board before the ship arrived in port, and if there had been no fresh cases of influenza for forty-eight hours, the sick were removed to hospital and after nominal rolls had been prepared giving the name and destination of each man, the troops were allowed to proceed by train. The nominal rolls were sent to the LGB for despatch to the MOH of the districts to which the demobilised men were proceeding. If there were any fresh cases within twenty-four hours, the whole of the troops, after the sick had been removed to hospital, were detained at camps adjacent to the ports, where they were kept under strict medical supervision for forty-eight hours. All healthy men were then allowed to proceed to dispersal camps or commands. In the cases of troops arriving for demobilisation on ships also carrying civilians, special difficulties were experienced in dealing with contacts owing to the port medical officer allowing the civilians to proceed to their destinations.[43] Many Irish troops would have returned on the mail boat to Kingstown or other ports on boats shared with civilians. Like the arrangements for transporting troops by rail, these measures would seem to have limited the opportunity for the spread of influenza from returning soldiers to the civilian population, but once again, more work needs to be done on demobilisation before we can know how well these measures were applied in practice.

Different arrangements applied to casualties of war: these were transported home on hospital ships, to Dublin in the first instance. From there, they would be distributed to appropriate hospital facilities under the control of the army around the city or in other towns. Sick soldiers were transported to facilities outside Dublin on two specially equipped army ambulance trains, one serving towns along the Northern Line to Belfast, and the other serving the south, including the Curragh military hospital and Cork.[44]

Local Government Board's response

Newspaper reports and personal accounts of Spanish influenza tell of the dread which accompanied it; the unpredictability of the disease and its apparent targeting of young healthy adults, the inability of contemporary medicine and science to treat it or explain it, and the association with the horrors of war, all fed into this fear. Charles Rosenberg, arguing that an epidemic is by implication frightening, says that fear and anxiety create an imperative need for reassurance.[45] The LGB did not appear to understand this need for reassurance, plainly displayed through the provincial and national press in constant calls from medical doctors, members of the BOGs and crusading journalists for the board to show leadership during the crisis. There was no public pronouncement from the *de facto* head of the board, vice-president, Sir Henry Robinson or the successive Chief Secretaries Shortt and Macpherson who were also ex-officio members of the board. The extent of the Board's direct connection to the people during the epidemic was its memorandum on influenza, which is unlikely to have been of much influence given the failure of the provincial press and some of the Dublin dailies to refer to it. Throughout the epidemic, the LGB kept a low profile, preferring, it seemed, to deal with the BOGs and local authorities through its inspectors there was one notable exception, an interview by an unnamed LGB source with an *Irish Times* journalist.[46] The only reasonably visible face of the Board during the crisis, in Leinster, was its inspector T.J. Browne, who advised local authorities on adding influenza-pneumonia to the list of notifiable infectious diseases, and who also suggested to the Dublin Board of Guardians quite early in the second wave that they ought to employ more doctors in places where medical officers might need help to tend the influenza victims.[47] Browne, according to the *Evening Herald* of 31 October 1918, had conducted an official tour of Leinster and discovered flu raging everywhere, but particularly in Wicklow, Wexford and Kildare. In the same report he pointed out that in Ireland the authorities were handicapped by their powerlessness to enforce measures to prevent the spread of infection, such as the closure of all places of public assembly.[48]

The Irish LGB's attitude towards its perceived responsibilities was not unique. Similar charges were laid against the LGBs for England and Wales during and after the influenza pandemic, and against the LGB for Scotland during the cholera epidemics of the nineteenth century. Niall Johnson noted that the LGB for England and Wales showed 'no desire ... to apply any controls to prevent the spread of influenza', leaving any such measures to the discretion of the local authorities; some might argue that under sanitary legislation this was an appropriate delegation, as they were the primary structures in place for dealing with epidemics and public health.[49] While the usual explanation for this was a policy of laissez-faire, there be may other reasons: first of all, that the composition of the LGBs and of their staffs shaped their attitudes towards dealing with the sick during an epidemic, particularly the sick poor; and secondly that the membership of the Boards included people whose expertise and interests were in other fields than public health. The Irish Board was ultimately answerable to the Irish Establishment, whose chief officers in 1918 were Lord Lieutenant John French and Chief Secretary Edward Shortt (the ex-officio nominal head of the LGB), both appointed to take a tough line with the growing Irish political crisis and to introduce conscription; instead, the more immediate crisis they encountered was an influenza pandemic (at a time when medical services were suffering from staff shortages because of the war) and public health was outside their area of expertise. Many of the staff positions within the Custom House could almost be regarded as hereditary, the preserve of certain families within a Protestant middle class, so concepts and philosophies of dealing with epidemic disease and with the sick poor might have changed little over generations.[50]

Criticism of the LGB's handling, or more correctly, lack of handling, of the epidemic, came from several different quarters. Some criticism was clearly political in origin, coming from Sinn Féin's advanced nationalists and their propaganda team. Other criticism came from newspaper journalists, including some working for Unionist or pro-establishment newspapers, from the BOGs (who at this stage mostly leaned towards nationalism) and from people working in healthcare, who were faced with not only a public health crisis but also with the sense that their work was being hampered by their masters' ineptitude. Rafferty, the MOH referred to in Chapter 2, was one of the more vocal doctors on the issue. After the first wave had subsided, he called on the LGB to take measures to guard against a reappearance of the epidemic with the change of weather in autumn, but complained that his warning was ignored. During the second wave, he complained that the supply of vaccines was not plentiful enough. He suggested that the LGB should provide local depots where residents could get vaccinated, as the best way to prevent the continued spread of influenza. Vaccination was a proven preventive against infection, he said, and also gave people confidence they were more immune to attack.[51] *Evening Herald* journalists were among the sterner critics of the LGB, backing up their case for more intervention with examples of strategies devised by health authorities in the United States and accusing the Board of a policy of laissez-faire towards the crisis. The *Herald*'s leader writer cited US campaigns for dealing with the scourge: prompt closure of theatres, picture houses and schools and giving the public warning of the dangers of infection posed by large gatherings. They had also mobilised 4,000 nurses to care for the sufferers, and had moved nursing units from city to city as urgency required.[52]

> We are also, we think, justified in this connection in asking the question: whether our Public Health Authorities are doing everything possible to combat this malignant and widespread disease? We have already alluded to the vigorous campaign organised by the corresponding authorities in New York and other American cities. Up to the present, we have not heard of action along similar lines taken by our own public health authorities ... A policy of drift or an attitude of *laissez faire* in such an emergency cannot be tolerated, and the battle against disease must be organised on systematic and thorough lines. To what extent this is being done at the present moment we are unable to say.[53]

Two days later, as the disease continued to worsen in Dublin city, the *Herald* leader writer felt it necessary to reiterate their criticism of the authorities:

> In the first calling to the serious visitation of the mysterious disease which is claiming a very heavy toll of victims in Dublin, as elsewhere, the 'Herald' warned the Health Authorities that: 'a policy of drift or an attitude of *laissez faire* in such an emergency cannot be tolerated, and the battle against disease must be organised on systematic and thorough lines. To what extent this is being done at the present moment we are unable to say. But the urgency of the matter must be apparent to everyone ... One must be careful not to create undue alarm, but we must again urge our health authorities to take urgent action and all necessary measures to grapple with what is generally recognised as a very serious scourge of humanity.'[54]

Even papers that were generally uncritical of the establishment could not contain their puzzlement at the Government's perceived inaction. The usually pro-establishment *Kildare Observer* decried the Government's 'attitude of almost supineness towards a malady which has been the cause of a tremendous death toll. This government

inertia ... should not be allowed to go on without at least a serious effort being made in the battle with the disease'.[55] The *Dundalk
Democrat*, alluding to Trinity College's Professor Culverwell's claim to
have developed an effective influenza vaccine, reported that 'Professor
Culverwell offers to take steps to enable any medical man communicating with him to obtain a supply of the vaccine, and suggests
that all the bacteriological laboratories ought to be employed in
making stocks of vaccine. What are the public health authorities at
the Custom House doing about this?'[56]

An *Irish Times* interview with an unnamed medical source in the
LGB was a defensive explanatory response to criticism. The official
said that through its inspectors, and by the issuing of certain advice
and instructions, the board had done everything it could possibly do.
The Irish LGB, he claimed, had taken the same actions as those taken
by the English LGB; where powers did not enable them to order
certain courses of action they issued advice when the circumstances
appeared to merit it.[57] This source mentioned that a recent memorandum on influenza contained the 'most up to date scientific information'. Fusty and convoluted, the memorandum (published by the
Irish Times on 30 October) contrasted sharply with the practical
advice contained in the bullet point memorandum issued by the
Dublin Corporation Public Health Committee. The LGB's memorandum read as follows:

> In the present limited state of knowledge with regard to influenza,
> the advice which it is possible to give the public both as to treatment
> and as to preventive measures differs but little from that which is
> appropriate to other infectious diseases. Early recognition of the dis-
> ease was important, as it was probable that the infection was chiefly
> spread during the initial stages of an attack. It is very desirable that
> any person suffering from a fever, with or without catarrh, should at
> once obtain medical advice, and should remain in bed at home until
> quite well. The use of boracic and weak saline solution for the frequent
> douching of the nasal passages is recommended. Infection is scattered
> by the act of sneezing or coughing, and this risk may be minimised by
> the habitual use of a handkerchief, which afterwards should be boiled,
> or if of paper, burnt. General disinfection of premises after influenza
> is not required, but a thorough washing and cleansing of rooms and
> their contents and washing articles of clothing used by the patient is
> advisable. No standard vaccine is available for the treatment of influ-
> enza, and although in cases of primary pneumonia and bronchitis,

treatment with a vaccine prepared from the particular pneumo-coccus or other organisms present in the secretions of the patient has sometimes been found useful, no such treatment can be recommended for the pulmonary complications of influenza. The inhalation of certain essential oils and doses of drugs, such as quinine or cinnamon, have been adopted for purposes of protection, but cannot be said with certainty to ensure freedom from attack. The gargling of the throat night and morning with a solution of one in 5,000 permanganate of potassium in water containing 0.8 per cent of common salt is useful as a preventive measure. It should also be drawn up through the nostrils and ejected by the mouth. Complete ventilation of each occupied living room and bedroom is recommended, as well as the avoidance of overcrowding in dwellings, the temporary discontinuance of public meetings and entertainments; the observance of strict cleanliness in the person, the home, and the workshop; abstention from indiscriminate spitting, and active realisation by any person suffering from influenza or catarrh that he may convey the infection to others, with possibly fatal results.[58]

The LGB's annual reports for the year of the crisis and the following year give further clues as to the board's mindset. In the report for the year ending 31 March 1919, which covers most of the epidemic period, the Board appears determined to take ownership of the hard work that its MOHs had done during the epidemic, either omitting to mention or glazing over the obstacles the board persistently placed in their paths. It lists the actions it had taken to combat the epidemic:

> For the general guidance of the public we issued advice and suggestions, founded on experience of epidemics of disease, for avoiding infection, and for dealing with attacks when developed ... We afforded local authorities all possible facilities for the employment of additional medical and nursing assistance, and recommended county councils that they might set free their tuberculosis officers to undertake the functions of district medical officers, where need existed.

Having considered adding influenza to the list of notifiable diseases, the Board concluded that notification would not be likely to be effective in checking the spread of the infection, because of the short incubation period, the difficulties of differential diagnosis, the varied forms which the disease assumed and its infectivity in the early stages of attack. This view, they said, was shared by authorities controlling public health administration in other portions of the UK. They did in fact decide to advise the extension of the Infectious Disease (Notification) Act 1889 to include septic pneumonia and this course was adopted in a number of districts. Concerned about the introduction of exotic infectious diseases as a result of the demobilisation and return of troops, the Board had introduced the Public Health (Ireland) (Pneumonia, Malaria, Dysentery, etc.) Regulations, 1919, prescribing the notification of malaria, dysentery, trench fever, acute primary pneumonia and acute influenzal pneumonia. Not only had the influenza epidemic taught the board how easily certain diseases could spread, it had drawn attention to the threat posed by the various types of pneumonia, which was, in 1918, a major killer quite apart from the influenza epidemic. Making the regulations, the LGB expressed the hope that the notification of cases of pneumonia would be followed by investigations of the conditions under which pneumonia had occurred and an increased knowledge of its natural history.[59] As well as covering notification, the regulations also empowered local authorities to provide medical assistance for pneumonia patients. The LGB said it had followed closely all available information about prophylactic vaccine treatment, but that it had not been convinced of its efficacy in conferring immunity: 'The general result of the experience of the past epidemic may be fairly summarised by saying that in order to cope successfully with future invasions further progress in the scientific determination of the microbic causation of the disease seems essential.'[60]

The Board's praise for the various Poor Law medical employees implied a situation far more under control and under their charge than the picture presented by the newspaper reports and in the BOGs' discussions of the crisis. The Board wrote of how the widespread prevalence of the disease at times made it difficult to provide medical attendance for all patients who needed treatment in their own homes:

> Medical Officers worked with most commendable zeal, and Guardians spared no expense in their endeavours to secure extra medical assistance. The supply of doctors, for temporary duty was limited mainly due to the large numbers of practitioners then serving with the forces, but the available resources were fully utilised.[61]

The annual reports point out that county councils released their tuberculosis medical officers for Poor Law work. In a few unions, the guardians, with the sanction of the LGB, appointed temporary district nurses to care for influenza patients.[62] The Board's praise is checked by reprimands over what they perceived to be excessively high fees demanded and paid to temporary district nurses and medical officers.[63]

The Board's reports on many of these issues, as well as the various issues to do with notification, could be at best described as disingenuous, and at worst as an attempt to whitewash what was in reality an organisational shambles, which was only rescued by the goodwill and devotion to duty of the Poor Law MOHs. With most of the issues, the decisive action they claimed was actually taken either in the third phase or after the epidemic had passed. For example, their circular withdrawing the prohibition on filling dispensary vacancies which had been in place since November 1915 was only issued on 9 April, 1919, as the epidemic was beginning to decline, and five months after the war it was introduced for had ended.[64] During the year from April 1919 to March 1920, the board arranged for a free supply of an influenza vaccine composed of the influenza bacillus (which the board also called Pfeiffer's bacillus) combined with strains of pneumococcus and streptococcus to doctors, with the proviso that they should keep careful records. By the time the vaccine arrived, all waves of the epidemic had passed.[65]

The annual reports of the LGB for the year spanning the influenza epidemic and for the subsequent year strive to create the impression of a caring and benevolent public body whose capable servants and well organised public health system had fought valiantly and coped for the most part successfully with a formidable enemy. The reports praise the medical officers of health, and even claimed that they had acceded to demands for increased fees with magnanimity, taking cognisance of the unusual circumstances, when the evidence from the BOGs' reports shows that the LGB quibbled constantly over fees. Deliberate destruction of LGB records during the revolutionary period, when the Custom House headquarters of the LGB – loathed by the revolutionaries – was burned, make it difficult to assess what deliberations the Board had on the influenza crisis. It is perhaps a measure of the level of interest the LGB had in the epidemic, and in their confidence of their own ability to deal with it, that the long-serving permanent secretary and vice-president of the Board,

Sir Henry Robinson, omitted to mention this last great challenge his board faced before its abolition, in his 1923 autobiography, even though he stated his intention to use the book to document the 'final eventful years of local government administration', and talked about the perpetual pressure that has always been the lot of the LGB.[66] After its abolition Robinson went to live in England out of concern for his personal security. It would be difficult to deny that the Board's failure to publicly take charge of the influenza crisis added in no small measure to the unpopularity of the LGB, and that it was part of the process in which the authority of the administration was undermined. The telling omission of the Board's handling of the Spanish influenza crisis from Robinson's autobiography may be silent testament to his sense of failure.

Notes

1 Emmet O'Connor, *A Labour History of Ireland, 1824–2000* (Dublin: UCD Press, 2011), pp. 102–273; Ruth Barrington, *Health, Medicine and Politics in Ireland 1900–70* (Dublin: Institute of Public Administration, 2000), p. 68.

2 Ibid., pp. 73–4.

3 P. Martin, 'Ending the pauper taint: medical benefit and welfare reform in Northern Ireland, 1921–39', in Virginia Crossman and Peter Gray, *Poverty and Welfare in Ireland 1838–1948* (Dublin: Irish Academic Press, 2013), pp. 223–36.

4 For a thorough discussion of hospital provision in Ireland and Britain in this era see Donnacha Seán Lucey and Virginia Crossman, eds, *Healthcare in Ireland and Britain from 1850: Voluntary, Regional and Comparative Perspectives* (London: Institute of Historical Research, 2015). Circumstances of specific hospitals during the pandemic are discussed in Chapter 6.

5 See interviews with R.B. MacDowell, Olive Vaughan and Dr James Walsh in Chapter 7, and D.W. Macnamara, 'Memories of 1918 and "the flu"', in *Journal of the Irish Medical Association* (October, 1954), xxxv, no. 208, p. 304.

6 Thomas Hennessy, FRCSI, DPH, 'Medical reform for Ireland', *British Medical Journal*, i, no. 3039 (29 March 1919), pp. 48–50.

7 Peter Martin, 'Medical and public health ending the pauper taint: medical benefit and welfare reform in Northern Ireland, 1921–39, in Virginia Crossman and Peter Gray, eds, *Poverty and Welfare in Ireland 1838–1948* (Dublin: Irish Academic Press, 2013), pp. 223–6.

8 *Medical Press*, 12 February 1919.

9 James Kelly noted his grandmother's reluctance to go the Belfast Union workhouse hospital for treatment when she got influenza. See Chapter 7.

10 *Ministry of Health Act, 1919. Report of the Irish Public Health Council on the Public Health and Medical Services in Ireland,* 1920 (cmd 761).

11 See Chapter 3 for an assessment of the morbidity of the disease based on available statistics.

12 Hennessy, 'Medical reform for Ireland'.

13 A guinea was 21 shillings, or one pound and one shilling (£1.05 in contemporary money).

14 *The Nationalist,* 9 November 1918. Minutes of the Dublin Union Board of Guardians meetings for October and November 1918.

15 Minutes of the Naas Board of Guardians meeting on 10 December 1918; personal communication with Joan Gogarty, Main St, Naas; the experience of the Gogarty family illustrates the danger influenza posed to those who worked in the retail trade.

16 Minutes of the Naas Board of Guardians meeting on 10 December 1918; Dr Morrissey's letter is dated 25 November 1918.

17 Minutes of the Dublin Union Board of Guardians meetings for October and November 1918.

18 See reports throughout the two months in Carlow's *Nationalist,* the *Dundalk Democrat,* the *Kilkenny People,* the *Enniscorthy Echo,* the *Evening Herald,* the *Enniscorthy Guardian,* the *Kildare Observer,* the *Leinster Leader,* the *Meath Chronicle,* the *People;* the Dublin BOGs' minute books for October and November 1918.

19 *The Nationalist,* 9 November 1918.

20 See, e.g., V. Crossman, *Politics, Pauperism and Power in Late 19th Century Ireland* (Manchester: Manchester University Press, 2006), p. 3. Crossman notes the tensions between the LGB and BOGs that were increasingly nationalist in composition, suggesting that boards exercised a certain amount of autonomy in their administration of the Poor Law at local level.

21 H. Robinson, *Further Memories of Irish Life* (London: H. Jenkins, 1924), pp. 185–8.

22 See, e.g., John Wylie, 'The Irish dispensary doctor', *British Medical Journal,* 26 September, 1891; Digby Ffrench, 'The Irish Dispensary Doctor', *British Medical Journal,* 31 December 1898.

23 *The Medical Press,* 12 February 1919; *British Medical Journal,* supplement to the *British Medical Journal,* 29 March 1919; *British Medical Journal,* 6 September 1919.

24 Irish supplement to the *Medical Press,* 20 November 1918.

25 *British Medical Journal,* 6 September 1919.

26 Forty-eighth annual report of the Local Government Board for Ireland.

27 *Evening Herald*, 26 October 1918.

28 See Chapter 2 for examples of Cameron's advice.

29 *Evening Herald*, 10 October 1918.

30 *Irish Times*, 14 October 1918. See also Kathleen Lynn's diaries in the Royal College of Physicians of Ireland Heritage Centre and Thomas J. Morrissey, *Laurence O'Neill (1864–1943): Patriot and Man of Peace* (Dublin: Four Courts Press, 2014), p. 124.

31 Issues to do with influenza and the nationalist movement will be discussed in Chapter 8.

32 *Evening Herald*, 23 October 1918.

33 *Irish Times*, 2 November 1918.

34 *Report upon the state of public health in the city of Dublin for the year 1919, by Sir Charles Cameron* (Dublin, 1920).

35 Dublin Corporation reports and printed documents, i, 1919, p. 587, 'Report of the Public Health Committee re hospital accommodation for influenza-pneumonia cases.'

36 *Irish Times*, 26 February 1919.

37 Kathleen Lynn diaries, 3 March 1919, Royal College of Physicians of Ireland.

38 *Nationalist*, 'The Eye on the Past No 769', personal communication with the author, Frank Taaffe, date of publication unknown.

39 *Report of the National Health Insurance Commission (Ireland) on the administration of national health insurance in Ireland during the period November, 1917, to 31 March 1920* (1921), xv, cmd 1147.

40 D. Ann Herring and Lisa Sattenspiel, 'Death in winter: Spanish flu in the Canadian Sub-arctic, in Howard Phillips and David Killingray, eds, *The Spanish influenza Epidemic of 1918–19: New Perspectives* (Abingdon: Routledge, 2003), pp. 156–72.

41 See, e.g., Patricia Marsh, 'The war and influenza: the impact of the First World War on the 1918–19 influenza pandemic in Ulster', in Ian Miller and David Durnin, eds, *Medicine, Health and Irish Experiences of Conflict, 1914–45* (Manchester: Manchester University Press, 2016), p. 34. *Aicid*, an Irish language documentary on the pandemic in Ireland made by Arkhive Productions for TG4 and BBC NI, has placed a strong emphasis on the role the rail network played in spreading the disease; *Aicid*, produced by Mary Jones, TG4 and BBC Northern Ireland, screened November 2008, June 2009.

42 Great Southern and Western Railway secretary's office files, annual report of the transport manager for 1918, GSWR Files 3027- 3078, Irish Railway Records Society, Heuston Station, Dublin.

43 Major-General Sir W.G. MacPherson, Colonel Sir W.H Horrocks, Major-General W.W.O. Beveridge, *Medical Services: Hygiene of the War,*

History of the Great War Based On Official Documents, I (London: HMSO, 1923), pp. 334–6.

44 National Archives: WO35/1794. Call for historical review of medical work in the Irish command during the war period. The information was collated for inclusion in the *Medical History of the War*.

45 Charles Rosenberg, *Explaining Epidemics and Other Studies in the History of Medicine* (Cambridge: Cambridge University Press, 1992), p. 294.

46 *Irish Times*, 2 November 1918.

47 Dublin Union BOG minutes, microfilm MFGS 49/091, file no BG 79/A82 National Archives, Dublin. The Dublin Union BOG minutes for 9 October 1918 documented a telephone message to the clerk of the union from the LGB inspector Dr T.J. Browne, noting that he recently visited the Grand Canal dispensary and thought that there was a possibility the medical officers would be unable to cope with the outbreak; he suggested the relieving officers should be authorised immediately to appoint medical officers to assist if medical officers could not visit all their patients. The Dublin Guardians approved his suggestion.

48 *Evening Herald*, 31 October 1918.

49 Johnson, *Britain and the 1918–19 Influenza Epidemic: a Dark Epilogue*, pp. 126–7.

50 F.J.M. Campbell, *The Irish Establishment, 1879–1914* (Oxford: Oxford University Press, 2009), pp. 86–7.

51 *Irish Times*, 30 October 1918.

52 *Evening Herald*, 21 October 1918.

53 *Evening Herald*, 21 October 1918.

54 *Evening Herald*, 23 October 1918.

55 *Kildare Observer*, 26 October 1918.

56 *Dundalk Democrat* and *People's Journal*, 26 October 1918.

57 *Irish Times*, 2 November 1918.

58 *Irish Times*, 30 October 1918.

59 *Forty-seventh annual report of the Local Government Board for Ireland.*

60 Ibid.

61 *Forty-seventh annual report of the Local Government Board for Ireland*

62 *Forty-seventh annual report of the Local Government Board for Ireland.*

63 *Forty-seventh annual report of the Local Government Board for Ireland*, p. 27.

64 *Medical Press*, Irish supplement, 9 April 1919.

65 *Forty-eighth annual report of the Local Government Board (for England and Wales), 1918–1919* (1920), xxiv, cmd 413, p. 40.

66 Sir Henry Robinson, *Memories Wise and Otherwise* (London: Cassell, 1923), p. xi.

5

The doctors' view: medical puzzle, politics and search for cures

From the beginning, this disease puzzled and frightened the public and medical experts alike. Public fears were imbued with a nervous tension informed by the background knowledge of the horrors of the First World War, of which this strange and overwhelming disease was an almost inevitable and often forecast sequel. For those working in the medical sphere, this disease challenged their expertise and tested their own confidence in advancements in medicine and their recently acquired and expanding knowledge of bacteriology. As with every outbreak of infectious disease, there were three critical questions to be answered: what was it, where did it originate and how could it be treated? This chapter will look at how debates on these questions unfolded in the Irish context.

Naming the 'mysterious malady'

The first question proved perplexing for a while. Irish newspapers, reflecting the opinions of the public and the medical profession alike, and following the international trend, were initially reluctant to name the disease, instead referring to it as a 'mysterious malady', a 'plague', a 'dread disease' or some other similarly non-diagnostic term.[1] The usually unmentioned undertone was that many expected a terrible disease to emerge from the gruesome war conditions. The conclusion of the 1870–71 Franco-Prussian War with a pandemic of smallpox was very much in the conscious memory of the public, the medical professions and the British Government; it was often alluded to in official reports and in the newspapers. Informed by this, and by other post-war disease events and other similar incidents, the government had established interdepartmental committees to cope with the expected increased incidence of infectious disease caused by the First World War, which was expected to increase significantly in the post-war period.[2] The leader writer of Wexford's *People* echoed the sentiments of many: 'A plague of some kind follows all great wars.'[3]

The historical basis for the healer's social role has been based on the sufferer's attempt not only to make a recovery but to find an explanation for their illness. Medical historian Charles Rosenberg has suggested that the healer's ability to diagnose and name the disease is an essential aspect of the healer's role: 'Even a dangerous disease, if it is made familiar and understandable, can be emotionally more manageable than a mysterious and unpredictable one'.[4] In the case of the 'new' disease which emerged in 1918, the medical profession was perplexed; confidence inspired by the development of the germ theory of disease and important developments in bacteriology which has enabled the formulation of vaccines to prevent or treat diseases that had seemed far more fearsome than the flu was shaken. Some of the discussion seemed to revert to the miasmatic concept of disease, with theories that the disease had come from vapours hanging over bodies left to rot in trenches on the European battlefields. The debate over naming expressed the anxieties of their profession. As they came to accept that this was influenza, albeit a rather extreme form of the disease, the fear seemed more manageable; there were fewer puzzled outcries.

Our contemporary medicine understands influenza as an acute and sometimes life-threatening viral infection of the respiratory tract, spread by sneezing or coughing. People become immune to an influenza virus after catching it, but influenza viruses are constantly changing. This happens either by 'antigenic drift', which are changes so small that most people previously exposed to a similar virus will still be immune, or by 'antigenic shift', which is a larger sudden change in an Influenza A influenza virus. Most people have little or no protection against the new influenza virus thus created, and so the risk of an influenza pandemic occurring is greatly increased. Such a shift took place in 1918, and subsequently in three other smaller pandemics, with the last one occurring in 2009.

Diagnosing influenza

Even today, influenza poses diagnostic difficulties. The World Health Organization advises that 'on clinical grounds alone it cannot be distinguished from other acute respiratory infection; laboratory tests are necessary.'[5] For the same reason, the Irish Health Surveillance Protection Centre refers to possible cases of influenza as 'influenza-like-illness' unless there has been a laboratory diagnosis of influenza. The centre advises that for a diagnosis of influenza a clinical picture compatible with influenza – sudden onset of disease, cough, fever greater than 38 degrees centigrade, with accompanying muscular pain and perhaps a headache – can only be confirmed with one of the following laboratory criteria for diagnosis: detection of influenza antigen, or influenza virus specific RNA, isolation of influenza virus, or the demonstration of a specific serum antibody response to influenza A or B.[6]

Back in 1918, the more obvious choice, influenza, was not initially accepted for several reasons, but principally because epidemic influenza had, as the medical textbooks agreed, high morbidity but not high mortality. As W.G. MacCallum, Professor of Pathology and Bacteriology at Johns Hopkins University put it in his *Text-book of Pathology* in 1918, 'For centuries it has been recognised that there is an epidemic disease, influenza or la grippe, which sweeps over whole continents, infecting nearly everyone, but causing few deaths.'[7] Influenza, according to MacCallum, was particularly marked by producing catarrhal inflammation of the upper air passages, fever and general prostration; although not particularly life-threatening, it was capable of causing a great variety of complicating consequences. This ailment was different: a mild disease in some people with the usual sore throat, fever and aches, in others it could become a killer within hours. It seemed to target young adults, whereas the groups more likely to succumb to influenza were the feeble, young and old. Haemorrhages, mostly nosebleeds, were common. The appearance of a mauvish tinge to the skin, termed heliotrope cyanosis, as the disease prevented the lungs from doing their job, seemed to be a symptom that was particularly alien to the normal symptoms of influenza; it alarmed not only the patient but watching family members and doctors. It happened as the tiny air sacs in the lungs, the alveoli, filled with blood and other body fluids, causing them to harden into a consolidated mass; as the alveoli filled, the amount of oxygen pumped into the blood was reduced, turning it from a healthy oxygenated red to a distinctly unhealthy shade of purple, which gave the skin a mauve colour.[8] This was one of the features of the new disease which led some observers to think that it resembled pneumonic plague, which kills most untreated patients within forty-eight hours of the onset of symptoms. As in cases of influenza, the pneumonic plague patient develops chills, high fever and often a severe headache after an incubation period of a couple of days; with plague, rapid breathing and shortness of breath are present. A rapid heartbeat (tachycardia) and a cough develop within a day or so, and the sputum becomes pink or red and foamy. Pneumonia can develop quickly, and septicaemia accompanied by with haemorrhages.[9] The heliotrope cyanosis often evident in people seriously ill with the 1918 influenza reminded people of the septicaemia associated with plague.

By the second wave in the autumn of 1918, the general conclusion was that the 'mysterious malady' was indeed influenza, in a severe form. There were still doubters, both in the newspapers and in the medical profession. 'Many question whether this can be called influenza', an *Enniscorthy Guardian* journalist wrote.[10] D.W. Macnamara, a newly appointed physician at Dublin's Mater Hospital in 1918, wrote forty years later that he remained unconvinced the disease was actually influenza, favouring instead a diagnosis of pneumonic plague. Having observed so many patients in the six worst months of the epidemic, he felt terms such as 'flu', 'la grippe', 'the Spanish flu', the 'black flu', and the 'falling sickness' (so called because so many people fell in the street on their way to or from work), all seemed unsatisfying or inadequate to describe it.

> The most striking thing … was the terrible prostration and toxaemia, and the revolting 'grogginess' that persisted for weeks, and sometimes even months in those lucky enough to recover, and somehow I was never satisfied in my own mind that the illness was influenza. To me, it was something much more terrible, and though I have never seen a case, I always looked on it as pneumonic plague. For it truly was a plague, a Black Death or what you will, but not influenza as we know it today.[11]

Dr Kathleen Lynn, Sinn Féin's director of public health, repeatedly registered her discomfort with the diagnosis of influenza, describing the outbreak among the republican prisoners in Belfast as a 'pneumonia plague'. In April 1919, her address to Sinn Féin's Extraordinary Ard Fheis referred to the 'so called influenza'.[12] Lynn's diatribe to the delegates about the aetiology of the disease was perhaps more a stylistic nod to Sinn Féin's propaganda campaign against the British Government rather than a real belief in the outmoded miasmatic theory of disease:

> There is no guarantee that we shall not have many more like outbreaks, for the factory of fever is still in full working order in Flanders – I mean the battlefield. The Germans were held up to us as inhuman monsters because they cremated their dead. The English and French have left millions of men and horses to rot unburied where they fell. Think a moment. Here the regulations require each single grave to be dug six-foot-deep for fear one corpse in decay injure the health of the community. A dead rat under the floor will render a room uninhabitable. In France and Flanders the poisonous matter from millions of unburied bodies is constantly rising up into the air, which is blown all over the world by the winds. Hence the influenza plague is universal … We cannot clean up the battlefields of Flanders, but we can talk about them and let the true cause be known.[13]

Clinical presentations and post-mortems

Although naming the disease as influenza helped to assuage some of the fears, the numbers of otherwise healthy people dying and the swift passage from well to dead for some continued to alarm all concerned. A man could rise from bed, have his breakfast, and leave for work. By lunchtime, his wife would be informed that he had died. It really could be that quick. Others recovered from the influenza attack, and resumed normal life, but died from post-influenzal pneumonia, heart attacks caused by the illness, or other complications. George Peacocke, physician at the Adelaide and president of the Royal Academy of Medicine in Ireland, told a meeting of the academy's section of medicine called to discuss the pandemic on 15 November 1918 that there was 'something akin to panic' among the public who had been 'unduly alarmed by the writings in the press'. The calling of an extraordinary meeting by the normally cautious medical profession to discuss the disease within a month of the onset of the second wave suggests that not only the public was alarmed: the doctors were worried too.[14] Dr James Walsh, retired deputy chief medical officer of the Department of Health, observed that when he was growing up in Co. Wexford (in a medical family) in the 1920s and 1930s, medical doctors still had an awful dread of the Spanish influenza; its apparent targeting of young people and the sudden onset of symptoms and transition to a severe stage alarmed a medical profession powerless to stop its path. D.W. Macnamara wrote of the terrible fear that prevailed during the epidemic, a fear which gripped people like a vice. 'No wonder. Once smitten with this disease there was no reasonable certainty of recovery.'[15] As a doctor, he said, one never knew with cases of the disease what was going to happen next:

> It was a depressing job ministering to patients with such a disease, with death at every corner of every ward, and it sometimes was a negative though very real comfort to look out of one of the windows facing towards Berkeley Road of a morning and watch the cavalcade of funerals trotting quietly and inevitable towards Glasnevin. At least one felt ... bad and all as it was in the Mater ... it was just as bad everywhere else.

Macnamara found it something of a consolation that other consultants and practitioners were no more successful with their therapies than the Eccles Street doctors. Dorothy Stopford Price's recall of assisting William Boxwell perform autopsies on influenza victims gives a sense of the urgency and excitement the disease provoked within medical circles:

> an interest [in post-mortems] inculcated in my student days by Professor William Boxwell. He was mad on post-mortems and I was acting as his clinical clerk in the November 1918 influenza epidemic. He tried to get a portion of lung from each victim of the 'black' influenzal pneumonia, and at 10 p.m. every night I biked down to the Mortuary, and with or without the aid of a night porter carried in about three corpses into the p.m. room, and stripped them ready and put them tidy afterwards; these were all surreptitious p.m.s and once or twice we got a fright when someone came to the door which was locked. I well remember nights when the rain came pelting down on the glass roof, and I alone inside trying to get the corpse into its habit and back to its bench; he often helped but was run off his feet and frequently had to leave at midnight on a call. He said the results of microscopic examination of the lung were disappointing, engorgement with blood obscured the picture.[16]

Peacocke told the Royal Academy of Medicine in Ireland (RAMI) meeting that he believed uncomplicated influenza of itself did not often cause death. In his view, the high mortality of the epidemic was due almost entirely to a high rate of secondary pneumonia and of streptococcal infection. While it was generally held that the causal organism of the influenza was the *bacillus influenzae*, he noted that many considered that some as yet undiscovered virus was responsible for the present epidemic. The symptoms he had seen were many and varied; severe cases, especially with pulmonary affections, frequently developed cyanosis, and usually resulted in death. Other features were laryngitis, delirium which could either be of a 'low muttering type' or a more violent type, mania which lasted even after the pyrexial period had passed, vomiting and albuminaria. Peacocke noted that the effects of influenza on the lungs also differed, and that many cases involved bronchitis or broncho-pneumonia. He considered the temperature chart a fallacious guide to the severity of the illness as in some severe cases there was hardly any fever. A sign full of omen was a fall in temperature without a corresponding fall in pulse and respiratory rate. Haemorrhages were another common complication, often in the form of nosebleeds, but sometimes they took a more serious form, such as brain haemorrhage. Tonsillitis and otitis media (middle ear infections) were not uncommon. He had not seen any influenzal meningitis. Peacocke said there was one outstanding form of the disease which deserved special attention:

> A patient, suffering at the time from a typical severe attack, suddenly becomes alarmingly ill … I have seen several such cases … one a young woman, 24, otherwise healthy, complained on a Wednesday night of being sick. Her temperature was slightly elevated. The next morning she was not so well, and fainted on getting out of bed. During the day her condition grew worse; she was removed to hospital, and when I saw her, at 7pm on Thursday evening, she was dying. Rales (crackles in the lung which could be heard with a stethoscope) were audible all over her chest; she was unconscious; her pulse was imperceptible, and she was coughing up fluid of the kind I have just described (rusty sputum). She died at 10pm the same evening.[17]

Macnamara also described different forms of the disease as it struck different organs of the body. There were gastric cases, cerebral cases and chest cases: 'very few non chest cases came to the Mater in my memory, and this may well have been due to the fact that such cases would in all probability have gone straight to a fever hospital as possible cases of enteric fever or of meningitis'. He noted that the most constant feature in the influenza patients he had examined – and he believed this number ran well into four figures – was the finding of moist rales at the lung bases, with usually only a little cough to account for them. 'The cough, alas, often came later, and with it a coalescing of all the little spots in the lung into patches of consolidation, which spread out until almost the whole lung was but one solid mass.'[18] He also wrote of its sudden onset, with many people collapsing at work or even in the street, and being well on their way to pneumonia by the time they reached the hospital.[19]

The clinical symptoms of the influenza reported by Irish doctors were broadly in line with those reported in other parts of the world. Levinson, a US Public Health Service clinician, reported observations taken at the Michael Reese Hospital of Chicago between 20 September and 31 December 1918. Of the 546 child and adult cases admitted, doctors chose fifty-five for a daily study of blood, urine and blood pressures, while the other cases the examinations were less frequent. They found that, for the most part, the onset of the disease was much the same, with the attack usually starting with a frontal headache; another constant symptom at the onset was pain or ache in the back. In addition, there were vague pains in the limbs, and often in the chest. Fever usually ranged between 103 and 104 degrees Fahrenheit. Some patients had a history of a chill at the onset; others first noticed a sore throat. Several spoke of pain in the lower-right side of the abdomen. Most of the patients did not have a runny nose, although they did sneeze a lot; some had nose bleeds. Many complained of pain in the trachea, lower down than the throat. By the third day, the cases could be divided into two groups – mild and severe. Mild cases were usually uncomplicated, and started to improve over the third day, although many complained of weakness for weeks afterwards. Severe cases were complicated by bronchopneumonia, by empyema (pus collecting in the pleural cavity between the outer surface of the lung and the chest wall) or by ear infections. Their temperature would remain high, and the cough would be unproductive and painful, which was usually the signal of broncho-pneumonia and the worsening of the condition, as the lungs hissed and sucked, trying desperately to fill with air the tiny alveoli which were already full of blood and mucous. In patients who were going to die, the temperature remained high, sometimes even as high as 109 degrees Fahrenheit. All fatal cases in the hospital during the study developed marked cyanosis; they then became unconscious and twitched frequently. They usually died between the sixth and the eleventh days of the disease, sometimes earlier.[20]

By 1918, the accepted causative organism of influenza was Pfeiffer's bacillus, also known as *haemophilus influenzae*, which was believed to have caused the Russian pandemic in the 1890s. Doctors searching for the causative organism of the 1918 epidemic expected to find Pfeiffer's bacillus, but the results were not conclusive. Some declared definitively that the disease was caused by a bacillus described by German bacteriologist Richard Pfeiffer in 1892, claiming to have isolated the bacillus in samples from sufferers. Captain John Speares, an assistant physician to the Adelaide Hospital Dublin, like Peacocke, noted in November 1918 that many medical workers agreed that the causative agent of this influenza was a bacillus similar to Pfeiffer's, and noted that the bacillus had been isolated from five cases of the first seven examined from flu sufferers in Howth. 'Since then the examination of over 150 sputa showed bacilli present, morphologically indistinguishable from Pfeiffer's, and in all probability genuine influenza organisms.' Speares, like Peacocke, noted that this influenza manifested in different forms, mostly respiratory, but sometimes gastro-intestinal. Like Peacocke, he thought the striking features were tendencies to various kinds of haemorrhage, albuminaria (which indicated damage to the kidneys), cyanosis and irregular temperature. Of the seven autopsies he had performed on influenza victims, two had recent extensive fibrinous pleural exudate on section of the lung. Some cases had extensive broncho-pneumonia; others showed definite areas of consolidation, especially in the right lower lobe, with a definite tendency to coalesce. Doctors at the Richmond Hospital examined sputum, nasal discharge, empyema fluid, lung tissue and heart's blood obtained post-mortem, but found no influenza bacilli. In all cases they found either pneumococci or streptococci, or both. The main type of pneumonia they found in the post-mortems was broncho-pneumonia.[21] Professor E.J. McWeeney also revealed that only a minority of the sputum specimens he had examined contained Pfeiffer's bacillus. In his experience the prevailing organisms were pneumococci, strepto-pneumococci, and micrococcus catarrhalis. Staphylococci were predominant in a few cases. He had not been able to arrive at any conclusion as to the micro-organism responsible for the primary influenza, but considered the pneumonia to be due to secondary infection with the above mentioned organisms.

Such findings dented the confidence of the medical profession in bacteriology, or at least in the then accepted bacteriological understanding of influenza. As influenza historians Howard Phillips and David Killingray have pointed out, little was known then about influenza and much of the research into the aetiology and epidemiology of influenza was focused in the wrong directions.[22] Influenza virologist Edwin Kilbourne has pointed out that the prevalence of secondary infections in influenza victims, including Pfeiffer's bacillus or *haemophilus influenzae*, led to the mistaken identification of it and other bacterial pathogens as causative agents. The causative virus of human influenza was not identified until 1933, and identifying the particular genetic structures of the 1918–19 pandemic proved impossible until recent years. Jeffrey Taubenberger, then chief of the Department of Molecular Pathology at the US Armed Forces Institute of Pathology, announced in October 2005 that he and his team had completed a ten-year-long quest to sequence all eight genes of the 1918 virus, and had identified it as an avian influenza virus strain. Almost simultaneously, Terrence M. Tumpey, a senior microbiologist with the US Centers for Disease Control and Prevention (CDC), announced that by using Taubenberger's gene sequencing he and his colleagues had created a live virus with all eight of the Spanish flu genes, in an effort to understand the biological properties that made the 1918 virus exceptionally lethal. The virus is being kept in a high-security government storage facility.[23]

Where did it come from?

Typically, a new form of influenza was expected to originate in Asia and move westwards; this influenza did not follow that pattern, and was at first widely believed to have originated in non-belligerent Spain whose press, being unrestricted by wartime censorship, reported freely on the illness of King Alfonso XIII, the Prime Minister, several Cabinet members and several thousand citizens of Madrid in May 1918.[24] However, it is now known that the influenza had already passed through army camps in the United States in March 1918. Historical and epidemiological data have so far proved inadequate to definitively assign a geographic point of origin, but historians and scientists continue to search and to debate the origin.[25] Some favour the theory that the influenza began in the United States in an army camp in Kansas in the spring of 1918, and was then carried back to Europe on board ship, its spread helped by overcrowding on the American troopships returning to the battlegrounds of Europe. In this camp are J.M. Barry, author of *The Great Influenza*, J.N. Hays in his work on human response to epidemics in 'Western' history, *The Burdens of Disease*, and Alfred W. Crosby, who continues to argue that while there were 'vague reports' of influenza-like illness in India, China and France in the early spring, contemporary documentary evidence points towards a starting point in early March in the United States.[26] Those arguing for an American origin doggedly refute the theory that the disease was caused by conditions in the First World War, while others firmly believe that the flu was cooked in the cauldron of the war on the European land mass. John Oxford and his colleagues estimate that there is sufficient evidence to suggest that the epidemic period began long before the outbreak in Kansas in overcrowded troop camps on the Western Front, and that the world war was indeed a contributing factor; the clustering of humans with the food to feed the armies – pigs and fowl – in close quarters, provided an ideal cauldron for the mixing required to create a reassortment of the influenza virus. Pigs, humans and birds are the main vectors for influenza. Doctors working at army camps at Étaples in France and Aldershot in 1915, 1916 and 1917 reported outbreaks of a disease they diagnosed as epidemic bronchitis, which presented with the heliotrope cyanosis that was later to become a feature in clinical diagnosis of Spanish influenza, and had a distressingly high mortality rate. Oxford uncovered a connection between Étaples and the American troop causation theory, and has suggested that American troops shipped back to the United States from the arena of war brought the influenza, or an earlier version, with them, thus confirming his theory that the flu had its origin in the theatre of war.[27]

The reluctance of some late twentieth- and twenty-first-century authorities to accept Oxford's locus of origin in the European arena of war is surprising, given that newspaper accounts, oral testimony and textbooks written in the immediate aftermath seem convinced that the flu came from the European battlegrounds. Several of the authors in F.G. Crookshank's collection of essays, *Influenza*, mention that diseases with similar symptoms were circulating from 1915 onwards in London and in France.[28] The British military reported outbreaks of influenza in many troop locations during the war years before the 1918 influenza came to be regarded as an epidemic. The British Expeditionary Force reported that it had outbreaks of influenza in France and Flanders in 1915, in Macedonia in 1915, 1916 and 1917, in the Dardanelles in 1915, in south-west Africa in 1914–15, in the United Kingdom in 1914 (6,047 admissions), 1915 (31,360 admissions), 1916 (36,072 admissions) and 1917 (28,980 admissions).[29]

The perspective from Ireland about the origin of the disease remained remarkably consistent throughout the epidemic period and after. Irish newspapers, as mentioned in previous chapters, made it clear they did not believe the disease originated in Spain. They, and most other authorities assumed, as Kathleen Lynn did, that it came from the war arena. Even among people interviewed for the purposes of this work, there was no suggestion that the disease had originated anywhere other than in the European battlegrounds and army camps. The disease had to enter Ireland, as an island, through the ports, and was perceived to have done so at the time. An early outbreak in May 1918 onboard the USS *Dixie* in Queenstown appears to have been contained. The east coast counties, whose ports had close ties with Britain, suffered the brunt of the first and second waves; Dublin, Howth and Kingstown were reported to be among the first areas to have large numbers of ill people, while the port towns of Dundalk and New Ross also suffered severe outbreaks. Although there is insufficient evidence to prove or disprove commonly held views that soldiers, whether demobilised or on leave, were a major vector in the diffusion of the disease, the constant movement of soldiers into Ireland during the period of the pandemic is almost certain to have been a factor, particularly in Dublin, which appeared to undergo reinfection in all three waves; the volume of civilian passenger traffic on the Irish Sea is also likely to have contributed to the spread. In the context of the movement of troops spreading the disease, it is worth remarking that Matthew Smallman-Raynor *et al.* note, in their spatial anatomy of this influenza in London and the county boroughs of England and Wales, that the population mixing associated with the phases of war (Wave I), demobilisation (Wave II) and peace (Wave III) did not fundamentally alter the structure of the diffusion processes by which influenza spread in the urban system of England and Wales.[30]

Treatment: vaccines, medical care, pharmaceutical and home cures

Throughout the epidemic, an energetic debate was conducted across the pages of newspapers and medical journals about whether or not vaccines were a useful adjunct to the efforts to contain and treat influenza. These articles often mention laboratories in Dublin city which were making vaccines, for instance, E.P. Culverwell's in Trinity College, Dublin, as well as Dr Crofton's laboratory in University College, Dublin. E.P. Culverwell's claims that his vaccine had been used successfully during the outbreak of the epidemic in Howth did not seem to impress the medical profession, who, for the most part, remained unconvinced about the efficacy of influenza vaccines.

Kathleen Lynn was an early and energetic proponent of vaccination. As soon as she was allowed off 'the run' on 31 October 1918, she opened up a centre in Charlemont Street to care for influenza sufferers and to vaccinate people against influenza, using a vaccine prepared by Dr Crofton at the National University Laboratory. She enthused that it was successful both as a preventive and as a curative measure, having used it on the influenza patients cared for in the Charlemont Street premises. About 14 per cent of those she inoculated caught the disease mildly, whereas about 44 per cent of the uninoculated caught it, many cases being very severe. 'My experience is that we have the preventative and the cure in our hands. If our race is to be saved in subsequent, frequently recurring outbreaks, inoculation must be systematically carried out on every man woman and child. Only thus will our people be saved.'[31] Others were more circumspect about approving the vaccine. Dr Charles McCormack, the medical member of the General Prisons Board, refused to supply requested vaccines to Clonmel Borstal Institution during a severe outbreak of influenza in the area on the grounds that the merits of vaccination for influenza 'is not yet placed on a sure footing so far as the general opinion of the medical profession denotes'.[32]

The prophylactic and curative attributes of influenza vaccines were the subject of an extensive debate at the November 1918 meeting of the RAMI; the broad consensus was that there was no consensus. George Peacocke, introducing the topic, described the value of influenza vaccine as a 'burning question at this time'. He had used the Trinity College vaccine in a few cases, but could not see any particular effect after using it. John Speares said that he began prophylactic treatments on 7 October; he did not favour the use of mixed vaccines of streptococcus and pneumococcus used in other countries but not extensively in Ireland. It seemed more logical to try to prevent the primary influenzal attack, and in any case it was difficult to regulate dosage and gauge resulting immunity when using a mixed vaccine. He thought rigid isolation was the most efficient prophylactic treatment. Speares believed that a vaccine of *bacillus influenzae* conferred some immunity if delivered in suitable doses. Dr Moorehead had a decided impression that as a prophylactic they were useful, mitigating the severity of the attack. He did not favour their use in severe cases. Dr O'Kelly had caught the disease while making a vaccine; he had heard good reports of a combined vaccine of pneumococci and micrococcus catarrhalis, but thought it too soon to make any conclusions about the use of vaccines until more data became available. Dr Nesbitt of the Richmond Hospital reported a brief but unfortunate personal experience of the vaccine as a prophylactic, as he contracted the disease within twelve hours of vaccination. The hospital had administered autogenous vaccines, mainly of the pneumo-streptococcus type, in the treatment of pulmonary cases, but he thought that on looking back over the case sheets their value was not convincing, though at the time they seemed to be effective. Dr Boxwell said that from the beginning he had regarded the more severe types as cases of profound septic intoxication. The typhus-like stupor, the haemorrhagic tendency of the complications, the severe albuminaria and haematuria, and the post-febrile delirium, all pointed in that direction, and called for a serum, which was available, rather than a vaccine. The evolution of the illness was too rapid for vaccine treatment to work, he thought. In the majority of cases patients were obviously getting over it, or were far too ill to call for a second dose. He had tried the vaccine, vaccinating half his cases only, but thought it had no effect. As regards the prophylactic use of the vaccine, he thought they were on surer ground. In general, prophylactic vaccination was scientifically sound, logical and based on plenty of analogous precedent. But he questioned whether the middle of a raging epidemic was the appropriate time to advocate wholesale vaccination, even supposing they had any real evidence that it would be effective. It was impossible to say who were already infected and who were free. In those already infected, vaccination was quite likely to precipitate an attack which they might otherwise have repelled. Dr Boxwell thought that the vaccination of contacts whole-sale in a household was unwise. The time for such inoculation was in the intervals of recurring epidemics, due care being taken to avoid possible sources of infection after the inoculation. Doses of reason-able size could then be used, at any rate without fear of doing harm. However, as it was impossible to foretell when the disease was going to flare up again in epidemic form, and the immunity conferred was in most cases short-lived, the value of prophylaxis in influenza was largely discounted. Dr Boxwell said he had seen one case in his own practice, and could vouch for two more, where rapidly fatal pneu-monia had followed from forty-eight to seventy-two hours after a prophylactic dose.[33] We do not know what was in Kathleen Lynn's vaccine, but given the content of other vaccines, and the opinion of other medical doctors working during this epidemic, it seems unlikely that the vaccine she was using would have had a preventive effect, and may even have caused further complications.

Medicinal treatment: strychnine or whiskey?

There was little consensus among the medical profession on the subject of the correct medicinal treatment for Spanish influenza, reflecting not only the difficulty of fighting an unknown enemy but also the wide variety of symptoms. Limited by lack of knowledge, they could only treat the influenza symptomatically. They seemed to throw the entire contents of their doctor's bag at the illness in the hope that something would work. George Peacocke admitted to his colleagues at the special RAMI meeting on influenza that he knew of no specific useful treatment. He usually employed sali-cylate of quinine as a routine, whereas aspirin appeared to relieve the headache. Like many other doctors, he considered keeping the bowels free and promoting sleep to be of great importance, so he prescribed calomel as a purgative, and trional or some preparation of opium for sleeplessness, a feature of this influenza in some cases. He considered that stimulants were required in most cases, and in some ought to be given freely; although he did not mention a spe-cific stimulant, strychnine was frequently used, as a stimulant, during the epidemic. John Speares used a similar selection of drugs to those used by Peacocke: calomel, oxygen, stimulants, salicylates and strychnine. He also recommended that stimulants such as strychnine were required in most cases and should be freely given.[34] While these were standard medical treatments at the time, it is worth noting that many of them have long since been abandoned by the medical sphere because of their toxic effect. The British Pharmaceutical Codex was amended in 1942 to document a number of quinine preparations which had been either withdrawn or modified following concerns over the toxicity of quinine; one of the modified preparations was Syrup of Phosphate of Iron, Quinine and Strychnine, also known as Easton's Syrup, which had the quinine content removed.[35] This syrup was extensively used by influenza sufferers in 1918–19, and was mentioned in communications between the GPB and the LGB to Dublin wholesale pharmacists Boileau and Boyd during the epidemic.[36] Quinine, widely used during the influenza epidemic to reduce fever, was available with and without prescription; it is now known to be a cardiotoxin and even small amounts can have toxic effects on the retina which may result in blindness; it can also cause convulsions, coma and respiratory arrest. The alarm expressed by Arthur Griffith's companions (see Chapter 8) when they discovered he had consumed an entire bottle of quinine tonic was well founded. Strychnine was used during the epidemic in syrups and also in injected form as a stimulant. Poisons expert Kent Olson advised that any dose of strychnine ought to be regarded as life-threatening.[37] Calomel, otherwise known as mercurous chloride, was a great stalwart of the doctor's bag, used extensively as a purgative and as an ointment until its toxicity was discovered.

A mixture of whiskey and hot water with, if available, sugar, was perhaps the most widely available and effective treatment for the symptoms of influenza, although the price of the spirit had been raised by an increase in duty in the spring of 1918.[38] The vapours eased congestion, and the drink itself eased the pain and promoted sleep. It had fewer side effects than many of the other influenza treatments, apart from the short term inebriation.[39] Whiskey was a regular part of the requisition orders for most institutions during the era, including workhouses and their infirmaries. However, some unions, particularly in the more Protestant areas in Ulster, objected to the provision of whiskey in workhouses and dispensaries on moral ground. Dr H.S. Murphy, MOH in the Lisburn Union, complained that he had been forced to give a severely ill influenza patient an injection of strychnine because the Union refused to supply the workhouse with whiskey on a matter of principle. Dr Murphy managed to get the Union to reverse their decision by stating his conviction that the one reliable drug to give a patient who got into a certain state was either brandy or pot-still whiskey, which contained valuable ethers that no other drugs contained.[40]

In the Mater, influenza patients were placed in the Fowler position, a semi-sitting position with the head of the bed raised. They were given a purge, some drug from the aspirin family, an expectorant mixture if they had a cough, stimulants, and to help rest at night, trional. Poulticing the chest with linseed meal was carried out as a routine in the pneumonic cases. D.W. Macnamara reported that it gave great relief from pain, had a remarkably uplifting effect on the patient's morale, and was always credited with the recovery if there was a recovery. He mentioned two other therapies popular at the time for grave cases: oxygen and injections of camphor in olive oil. Oxygen, in his view, was almost never used in time, as it was regarded as something that ought to be used only in the greatest possible emergency. The camphor treatment he described as 'the very nadir of therapeutic bolony'. Although he was instructed by his seniors to use it, he felt guilty that he had inflicted further pain and suffering on the helpless ill, and that they would have done much better if he had left them alone. Other popular treatments for influenza were quinine and the cough mixture senega; the latter he thought caused more harm than good as it upset already delicate stomachs; he considered that Pot. Iod. (potassium iodide) and Spts. AMM. Aromat. with Paregoric (anhydrous morphine) and Tinct. Digitalis to support the heart were valuable ancillaries. Some doctors, especially his older colleagues, favoured whiskey or brandy 'in heroic doses'. Alcohol, he suggested, had a good deal to recommend it, as it was 'probably no less worthless than any of the other nostrums, and at least its customers had a merry spin to Paradise'.[41]

Potions and folk remedies

Non-prescription medicines were in high demand, as people tried to self-medicate. As well as compounding regular medicines, pharmacists worked long hours to prepare huge quantities of tonics, cough medicines and poultices. The poultices were usually a mixture of boiling water and ground linseed, reputed to aid decongestion, enclosed in cloth and placed on the chest or throat.[42] As everybody searched for an effective treatment, journalists passed on tips to their readership. The *Irish Independent* observed that Major R.T. Herron, Medical Officer, Armagh Union infirmary, had suggested gargling with a solution of permanganate of potash as a useful preventive measure. Sir R. Winfrey, MP, a qualified chemist, recommended a prescription of thirty drops pure creosote, a half-ounce of rectified spirit, three-quarters of an ounce of liquid extract of liquorice, two drachms of salicylate of soda and twelve ounces of water, with the recommended adult dosage of two tablespoonfuls three times daily.[43] Many newspapers reported that people were carrying handkerchiefs doused in eucalyptus oil in front of their mouths as a preventive measure. Macnamara said that eucalyptus was uncommonly popular, and people all over Dublin in trams, trains and theatres would pull out a handkerchief to sniff the oil. He believed it was about as potent to repulse influenza as a black beetle would be to halt a steamroller.[44]

Newspapers typically carried a heavy advertising schedule of potions, fortifiers and pills to attract the business of the self-medicator. As the pandemic developed, products which had, for example, been advertised as good for dealing with the exhaustion or neurasthenia caused by the war now claimed to cure influenza also. These advertisements are useful gauges of the public interest in influenza, and suggest that manufacturers saw the disease as a commercial opportunity. Many carried a subtext that the reason why the epidemic had been able to take such a hold on the population was that the Great War had debilitated people. An advertisement for Phosferine is typical of that tone. It advised that the tonic be used to combat the lingering effect of flu, with commendations from Red Cross workers in Belgium and soldiers from different regiments to prove the point:

> These soldiers are convinced that it is a public duty to testify to the unfailing efficacy of Phosferine as a preventive of, and remedy for, the disastrous scourge of INFLUENZA now raging throughout the world. Phosferine stimulates the nerve centres to produce the extra vital force needed to prevent the perilous nervous collapse and exhaustion so peculiar to influenza epidemics.[45]

Other advertisements traded on the public paranoia of catching infection, and the desire to disinfect houses and places of work from the threat of germs lurking within. In the beginning of March 1919, at the height of the third wave of influenza, an advertisement preying on this paranoia appeared on the front page of the *Irish Independent*:

> Influenza in Ireland!!! The dread disease is back again all over the land. Don't be taken unawares, protect yourself, your household, your children, your office, your factory, against the death dealing GERMS. Get at once a DEODAR. See the illustration. Spray its contents regularly. A child can use it. All the doctors in the world cannot give as much safety from the 'Flu'. Factory managers in the interests of their whole organisation, should order a DEODAR outfit at once. SPECIAL OFFER TO IRELAND'S householders, just to prove the exceptional efficiency of this excellent invention. COMPLETE OUTFIT, including sprayer and Deodar, 10/6, post free. This offer remains open while we have Sprayers. The demand all over the whole of the UK is simply enormous. A special supply has been put by for readers of the Irish Independent by urgent request. Deodar Company Ltd, 6 Exchange Arcade, Manchester.

On 4 March 1919, the *Irish Independent* reported that Goodbody's flour mills in Clara, King's County (Offaly) were supplying large quantities of the beef extract Bovril to their workers. Beef extract – or beef tea – was considered to strengthen bodies as a defence against infection. Over 300 employees were sick, and two, a mother and son, had already died. Goodbody's, a Quaker family, employed three special nurses to assist the local doctor and nurses to treat the staff.[46] Not to be outdone by Bovril, their chief rival OXO advertised on the front page of the following day's newspaper that 'OXO fortifies the system against influenza infection', and quoting from an alleged communication received from a doctor:

> A cupful of OXO two or three times a day will prove an immense service as a protective measure. Its invigorating and nourishing properties are most rapidly absorbed in the blood, and the system is reinforced to resist attacks of the malady. It will be apparent that a strong, healthy person will escape contagion when the ill-nourished one will fall a victim, consequently, one's aim must be the maintenance of strength.[47]

Small producers advertised their influenza-combating products in the provincial papers. Readers of the *Enniscorthy Guardian* were urged to 'pour a little Cousins' lemonade into a saucepan and warm it, to provide the perfect drink for influenza sufferers'.[48] The International Pharmacy at 21 Dawson Street, Dublin, offered Ashmore's Pilocarpine Lotion, guaranteed to help people whose hair had fallen out during their convalescence from influenza.[49] A pharmacist in Gorey, James E. Cooke, claimed that his cod liver oil emulsion could protect against influenza, while other chemists advocated Dr J. Collis Browne's Chlorodyne as a remedy not only for influenza, but also for coughs, colds, asthma, bronchitis, diarrhoea, colic, neuralgia, gout, toothache, rheumatism, spasms, hysteria and palpitations.[50] In the years before false advertising became an offence, purveyors could be bold with their claims and make sales by preying on the fears and ignorance of their clients.

Dublin's only homeopathic chemist, Victor E. Hanna, of the Prescription Pharmacy at 70 Lower Mount Street, recommended, in his advertisements, the use of a homeopathic pillule of gelsemium to combat the disease, claiming that not one single case of influenza had yet been reported in which it had been taken as a preventative, and those who used it as a cure had also had their symptoms alleviated.[51] Homeopaths prescribe gelsemium as the 'glass coffin' cure for an influenza typified by cold feet. Homeopathy was widely used in America during the pandemic.

While sufferers sought the comfort that they were taking a fortifier or something to alleviate the symptoms, many authorities agreed that bed rest and good nursing were more likely to improve the chances of survival than medication. The ever-practical Sir Charles Cameron gave common-sense advice to sufferers: go to bed and stay there until well after the attack has passed, in order to prevent a relapse. Macnamara said that any serious case that survived was due to the nurses rather than the doctors and their medications.[52] Kathleen Lynn recommended that someone who contracted the disease should go to bed at once, take an aperient and follow a liquid diet.[53] She advocated basic good hygiene practice in her address to the Sinn Féin Extraordinary Ard Fheis. Lynn stressed the importance of avoiding cross-contamination; simple methods like ensuring each patient had their own mug and spoon, washed up separately from others. Plenty of fresh air helped to mitigate the symptoms and to prevent the infection passing to others. Good nourishment helped also. She suggested that the ill should be given milk, barley water and egg flip, while those in good health ought to fortify themselves with milk, butter, eggs, fresh meat, vegetables and porridge.[54]

Health complications caused by influenza

Surviving an attack of Spanish influenza did not necessarily mean a return to health: there was a vast array of recognised post-influenzal complications, some of which could kill a long time after an apparent recovery. Many of these occur after any influenza, whether seasonal or pandemic, but the enormous numbers of influenza sufferers in the 1918–19 pandemic also increased the numbers developing post-influenzal complications. Macnamara reckoned that for the millions who died during the pandemic from influenza or pneumonia, there were many millions more who died from complications.[55]

The disease often damaged the heart and lungs, and caused various types of nerve, eye and ear disorders. Cecil Kidd, a Belfast-based doctor and one of the few Irish medical professionals to show enough interest in the pandemic to write about it, noted that the post-influenzal consequences could include cardiac complications: a severe attack caused some patients to become permanent cardiac invalids. He also noted that there were vascular complications, of which vascular lesions and blood clots were the most common. The vein inflammation, phlebitis, also occurred, and intermittent leg pain due to toxic arterial injury was recorded. He had heard of deficient arterial tone as a cause of continued post-influenzal cardiac weakness. The cranial nerves were sometimes affected, causing disturbed or temporary loss of smell. Inflammation or atrophy of the nerves in the eye and ocular palsies occurred. Other complications Kidd had heard of in association with this influenza pandemic were Bell's Palsy, which manifested in the paralysis of one side of the face, transient or permanent deafness, the nerve disorders neuralgia and neuritis, and also headache, loss of memory, insomnia and neurasthenia.[56] Smith Ely Jelliffe documented a similar list of the many different forms of what he considered to be mental disturbance caused by pandemic influenza, ranging from simple fatigue to aphasia (loss of words), depression, mental confusion, influenzal hemiplegia (the complete loss of motor function in one side of the body), post-influenzal neurasthenia and psychoses. Jelliffe said that if one omitted syphilis, there was probably no infectious disease that gave rise to so many diversified types of mental disturbance ranging from simple fatigue to severe and debilitating mental illness.[57]

Many authorities believed there was a link between an almost contemporaneous epidemic of encephalitis lethargica and the Spanish influenza pandemic.[58] Epidemics of encephalitis lethargica (a swelling of the brain which makes one sleepy) have been associated, under various names, with severe epidemics of influenza as far back as the European influenza pandemic in 1580, according to Price and others. The disease, which often begins with an influenza-like illness with a high temperature, can result in the patient becoming progressively lethargic to the extent that he or she can lie still for days without moving a muscle, paying no notice to his surroundings, and excreting and urinating unheedingly. In 1916, Von Economo succeeded in transferring it into monkeys from humans by intracerebral inoculation; when the monkeys showed similar symptoms to the humans suffering from encephalitis lethargica, he had proved that it was an infectious disease. By performing autopsies, he found that there was a discernible pattern of brain damage in encephalitis lethargica victims; he theorised that depending on where the encephalitis lethargica bug had damaged the hypothalamus, the area of the brain known to control sleep, either too much or too little sleep resulted. French physician and pathologist Cruchet looked at a number of cases of soldiers in Verdun in 1915–16 suffering from sleeping sickness. At first he thought the syndrome as a result of mustard gas or some new chemical weapon, but he came to similar conclusions to Von Economo that the syndrome was caused an infectious disease. Price timed the outbreak associated with the Spanish influenza pandemic between 1917 and the 1930s.[59] Jelliffe suggested in the early 1920s that it was at epidemic levels all over the world since 1915. Kidd noted that a severe epidemic of encephalitis lethargica occurred in the first half of 1924.[60] It was sometimes confused with other diseases, including influenza and poliomyelitis. Some authorities have also posited that there was a connection between Spanish influenza and Parkinson's disease, and perhaps linking in encephalitis lethargica.[61] Recently Patricia Marsh has found that forty-two cases of the disease were treated in Belfast's Royal Victoria Hospital in between 1918 and 1923, perhaps connected with the influenza pandemic.[62] There may also have been an associated epidemic of Guillain–Barré syndrome, an ascending paralysis of the peripheral nervous system, first identified in 1916. Links between influenza and attacks of Guillain–Barré syndrome as a post-influenzal complication are now well known, particularly following the outbreak of an epidemic of the syndrome in the United States in the 1970s traced back to mass vaccination with an influenza vaccine rushed through the trial stages, when health authorities advised that an influenza epidemic posed an imminent threat.[63] The physical complications of Spanish influenza stayed with some survivors for the rest of their lives, which in some cases were shortened by those complications, as the testimonies of R.B. McDowell and Tommy Christian in Chapter 7 reveal.

This chapter has concentrated on exploring the debate about the identification and treatment of Spanish influenza in an Irish context, and looked at the main arguments about the origins of Spanish influenza. These arguments about the origin of the influenza have continued to shift as scientific knowledge moves on and as more historical data are uncovered, with each new discovery helping to form a more complete picture of the aetiology of a disease that is clearly easier to investigate using knowledge which has evolved significantly in the intervening years. The Irish debate about identification and treatment of the Spanish influenza virus touched on many of the universal themes about Spanish influenza, the dread of some terrible disease emerging out of a terrible war, the fear of the public and the medical sphere alike as it prostrated and killed, the desperate and ultimately futile search for vaccines and treatments, and the fascination the disease held for pioneering doctors who queried the limits of their own medical knowledge and their confidence in bacteriology, and sought to improve the answers.

Notes

1 European mainland newspapers were also reluctant to name the disease: see Wilfred White, 'The plague that was not allowed to happen', in Howard Phillips and David Killingray, eds, *The Spanish Influenza pandemic of 1918–19: New Perspectives*. (Abingdon: Routledge, 2003).

2 *Ministry of Health: Annual report of the chief medical officer, 1919–1920* (1920), xvii, cmd 978; the author attributes the smallpox reference to Prinzing's *Epidemics Resulting from Wars*. See also *Irish Times*, 31 October 1918.

3 *The People*, 16 November 1918.

4 Charles Rosenberg, *Explaining Epidemics and Other Studies in the History of Medicine* (Cambridge: Cambridge University Press, 1999) p. 310.

5 Niall Johnson, *Britain and the 1918–19 Influenza Pandemic: a Dark Epilogue* (Abingdon: Routledge, 2006), p. 19.

6 See the Irish Health Protection Surveillance Centre's website at www.hpsc.ie.

7 W.G. MacCallum, *A Text-book of Pathology* (London: Saunders, 1918), pp. 556–7.

8 Mark Honigsbaum, *Living with Enza* (Basingstoke: Palgrave Macmillan, 2009), pp. 24–5.

9 Robert Berkow, ed., *Merck Manual of Diagnosis and Therapy*, fourteenth edn (Rahway, NJ: Merck Sharp & Dohme, 1982), p. 110, and MacCallum, *A Text-book of Pathology*, pp. 551–2.

10 *Enniscorthy Guardian*, 9 November 1918.

11 D.W. Macnamara, 'Memories of 1918 and "the Flu"', *Journal of the Irish Medical Association*, xxxv, 208 (1954) p. 304.

12 Kathleen Lynn diaries, in the Royal College of Physicians. Kathleen Lynn, 'Report on the pandemic of influenza', Sinn Féin Ard Fheis (extraordinary), 8 April 1919, pamphlet in National Library of Ireland.

13 Ibid.

14 *Medical Press*, 1 January 1919.

15 Macnamara, 'Memories of 1918 and "the Flu"'.

16 Liam Price, ed., *Dr Dorothy Price, an account of twenty years fight against tuberculosis in Ireland*, priv. circ. (Oxford, 1957), p. 4. William Boxwell lectured in medicine at Trinity College, Dublin, and was appointed professor of pathology and bacteriology at the Royal College of Surgeons in 1918; *Dictionary of Irish Biography* http://dib.cambridge.org 3 February 2010. See also Anne Mac Lellan, *Dorothy Stopford Price, Rebel Doctor* (Newbridge: Irish Academic Press, 2014).

17 *Medical Press*, 1 January 1919.

18 Macnamara, 'Memories of 1918 and "the Flu"'.

19 D.W. Macnamara, 'The Mater–1914–1919', *Journal of the Irish Medical Association*, xlix, no. 293 (November 1961), p. 147.

20 A. Levinson, 'Clinical Observations on influenza with special reference to the blood and blood pressure, *The Journal of Infectious Diseases*, vol. 25, no 1, July 1919, pp. 18–27.

21 *Medical Press*, 1 January 1919.

22 Howard Phillips and David Killingray, eds, *The Spanish Influenza Pandemic of 1918–1919: New Perspectives* (Abingdon: Routledge, 2003) p. 6.

23 Mike Mitka, '1918 Killer flu virus reconstructed, may help prevent future outbreaks', *Journal of the American Medical Association*, ccxciv, no. 19 (2005), pp. 2416–9.

24 Beatriz Echeverri, 'Spanish influenza seen from Spain', in Phillips and Killingray, eds, *The Spanish Influenza Pandemic of 1918–1919*, pp. 173–90.

25 Jeffery Taubenberger and David Morens, '1918 Influenza: the mother of all pandemics', *Emerging Infectious Diseases*, xii, no. 1 (January 2006), pp. 15–22.

26 J.M. Barry, *The Great Influenza* (London: Penguin Books 2005). J.N. Hays, *The Burdens of Disease* (New Brunswick, NJ: Rutgers University Press, 2003). Alfred Crosby, *America's Forgotten Pandemic* (Cambridge: Cambridge University Press, 2003), pp. 21–5.

27 J.S. Oxford, A. Sefton, R. Jackson, W. Innes, R.S. Daniels and N.P.A.S. Johnson, 'World War I may have allowed the emergence of "Spanish" influenza', *Lancet Infectious Diseases*, ii (February 2002). Interview with J.S. Oxford, Dublin, 7 May 2010.

28 Crookshank, *Influenza*, passim.

29 T.J. Mitchell and G.M. Smith, *Medical Services – Casualties and Medical Statistics of the Great War*. From the series Official History of the Great War based on official documents (London: HMSO, 1931), p. 86.

30 Matthew Smallman-Raynor, Niall Johnson and Andrew D. Cliff, 'The spatial anatomy of an epidemic: influenza in London and the County Boroughs of England and Wales, 1918–1919', *Transactions of the Institute of British Geographers*, new series, xxvii, no. 4 (2002), pp. 452–70.

31 Kathleen Lynn, 'Report on the pandemic of influenza', Sinn Féin Ard Fheis (extraordinary), 8 April 1919, pamphlet in National Library of Ireland. Kathleen Lynn diaries, Royal College of Physicians in Ireland. See also Margaret Ó hÓgartaigh, *Kathleen Lynn – Irishwoman, Patriot, Doctor* (Dublin: Irish Academic Press, 2006).

32 GPB, 1918/6886.

33 *Medical Press*, 1 January 1919.

34 John Speares, 'Influenza', *Dublin Journal of Medical Science*, 3rd series, no. 146 (1918), pp. 253–8.

35 See www.rsc.org/delivery/_ArticleLinking/DisplayArticleforFree.cfm?. doi=AN943600054&JournalCode=AN

36 GPB, 1918/6460.

37 Kent Olson, ed., *Poisoning and Drug Overdose* (London: Appleton & Lange, 1990), pp. 257–8, 274–5. W.H. White, *Materia Medica* (seventh ed., London, 1902), explains the use of strychnine as a stimulant.

38 GPB, 1918/6460.

39 See Chapters 4, 7 and 8 for a further discussion of the use of whiskey during the influenza epidemic.

40 *Irish Independent*, 5 March 1919.

41 Macnamara, 'Memories of 1918 and "the Flu"', p. 304.

42 Telephone communication with a family member of Phillip Brady, who worked as a pharmacist at Kelly's Corner, Dublin, during the epidemic; further details with author.

43 *Irish Independent*, 4 March 1919.

44 Macnamara, 'Memories of 1918 and "the Flu"'.

45 *Irish Independent*, 8 March 1919.

46 *Irish Independent*, 4 March 1919.

47 *Irish Independent*, 5 March 1919.

48 *Enniscorthy Guardian*, 7 November 1918.

49 *Irish Times*, 6 January 1919.

50 *Enniscorthy Guardian*, 30 November 1918.

51 *Enniscorthy Guardian*, 30 November 1918.

52 Macnamara, 'The Mater – 1914–1919', p. 147.

53 *Irish Independent*, 18 October 1918.

54 RCPI heritage centre: Kathleen Lynn diaries. Lynn, 'Report on the pandemic of influenza'.

55 Macnamara, 'The Mater – 1914–1919', p. 147.

56 C.W. Kidd, 'Epidemic influenza: an historical and clinical survey.' MD thesis, Queen's University Belfast, 1933.

57 Smith Ely Jelliffe, 'The nervous syndromes of influenza' in F.G. Crookshank, ed., *Influenza: Essays by Several Authors* (London: W. Heinemann, 1922), pp. 351–77. See also Svenn-Erik Mamelund, 'The long-term impact of historical influenza pandemics on mental health 1872–1930', ESSHC Conference, Ghent, 15 April 2010.

58 See, e.g., P.P. Mortimer, 'Was encephalitis lethargica a post-influenzal or some other phenomenon? Time to re-examine the problem', *Epidemiology and Infection*, xxxvii, no. 4 (April 2009), pp. 449–55; F.G. Crookshank, 'Encephalitis Lethargica', *British Medical Journal* (28 June 1919), www.jstor.org/stable/20338007; and H.F. Smith, 'Epidemic encephalitis (encephalitis lethargica, Nona): report of studies conducted in the United States', Public Health Reports (1896–1970), xxxvi, no. 6 (11 February 1921), pp. 207–42, http://jstor.org/stable/4575888.

59 Frederick Price, ed., *A Textbook of the Practice of Medicine*, seventh edn (Oxford: Oxford University Press, 1947), pp. 1608–15. Molly Caldwell Crosby, *Asleep: the Forgotten Epidemic that Remains One of Medicine's Greatest Mysteries*, electronic edn (New York: Berkley Books, 2010).

60 Kidd, 'Epidemic influenza'.

61 See, e.g., George Moore, 'Influenza and Parkinson's disease', *Public Health Reports (1974–)*, pp. 79–80, and Crosby, *Asleep*.

62 Patricia Marsh, '"Sleepy sickness spread" encephalitis lethargica in Belfast', paper presented at Society for the Social History of Medicine conference, Canterbury, 8 July 2016.

63 Arthur Silverstein, *Pure Politics and Impure Science: the Swine Flu Affair* (Baltimore, MD: Johns Hopkins University Press, 1981).

6

Hospitals and other institutions: coping with crises

Institutions are characterised by a rigid focus on organisation and management which is underpinned by documentation. We expect them to have created detailed records. But regular users of Irish institutional records from this period are aware that some have been lost, or destroyed during the revolutionary period. Those that do survive often offer little to recreate a picture of how the institutions coped with this extraordinary disease phenomenon. Some institutions or their regulating authorities give only a passing nod to the pandemic in their reports; perhaps it did not affect their operations or was outside the regular blueprint for reporting. Official annual reports tend to follow the same outline and often little changes in the wording year after year. Others break away from the arid official language that typifies reports, as though the author understood that something extraordinary was happening and wanted to leave their record of it. These noteworthy exceptions can offer fulsome details of influenza's effects on institutions, as this chapter will show through a discussion of the correspondence between the GPB and their officers, and the keenly detailed journal reports from Clongowes Wood College, a Jesuit boarding school in Co. Kildare.

Despite the limitations of institutional records, a number of common themes do emerge. When the influenza pandemic struck, it disrupted normal operations. The funding crises that the hospitals faced perennially were already intensified by a sharp rise in inflation towards the end of the war. This further depletion of their resources made their funding situations acute; charitable hospital and Poor Law unions records from the period are replete with complaints about rises in costs of medicine and other provisions, as well as problems caused by the coal shortage. Many had given over beds normally available to treat the civilian population for the treatment of wounded soldiers. Rising costs and the fuel crisis affected all institutions.

The epidemic and public and charitable hospitals

The annual reports of the Board of Superintendence of Dublin hospitals are among the few sources that give quantitative evidence of what was happening in Irish hospitals during the pandemic. These reports provide statistical information on deaths and illnesses, including influenza and pneumonia, of patients in all Dublin hospitals receiving grants from parliament: the House of Industry Hospitals (Hardwicke fever hospital, Whitworth medical hospital and Richmond surgical hospital), Dr Steevens' hospital, Westmoreland Lock hospital, Rotunda lying-in hospital, Coombe lying-in hospital, Meath hospital, Cork Street fever hospital (officially the House of Recovery and Fever Hospital), Royal Victoria Eye and Ear Hospital, and the Royal Hospital for Incurables. During the calendar year from April 1918 to March 1919, Dr Steevens' Hospital treated 470 cases of influenza, of which only two died. Of a further fifty-eight cases of pneumonia, thirty, or over 50 per cent, died. In the Hardwicke fever hospital, 280 cases of influenza were treated, of which twenty-eight died; thirty-one cases of pneumonia were treated, of which eleven, or 31 per cent, died. Of the Meath hospital's 173 influenza cases, only seven died, but sixteen of the twenty-one patients treated for pneumonia died, or 76 per cent of the cases. Two patients awaiting eye surgery in the Royal Victoria Eye and Ear Hospital died from influenza. The Whitworth had seventeen cases of influenza, with one death, and two cases of pneumonia, both surviving. Cork Street was the largest fever hospital in the city; severe cases of influenza were removed from the Dublin Union workhouse infirmary, and it also took in army cases of infectious disease. It treated 708 cases of influenza, with 173 deaths, or 24 per cent of the hospital's total influenza cases; there were 143 cases of pneumonia, of which twenty-four died, or 17 per cent. Some 15.05 per cent of Cork Street's 2,349 admissions in the year to the end of March 1919 died, compared to 7.78 per cent of the 2007 admissions for the following twelve months. The average annual admissions since it opened in 1802 had been 1380.[1] Cork Street's medical superintendent John Marshal Day wrote in his annual report the following year that it was sad to see how many of the pneumonia deaths were of former soldiers, 'whose resistance had been lowered by the hardships of war service'.[2] It is difficult to advance a convincing explanation for the variations in the success rate in treating influenza between the hospitals without more information as to how doctors in the different hospitals distinguished between cases of influenza and of pneumonia, and without knowing other factors, such as the methods of nursing care, the treatments, the levels of isolation and visiting policies during the pandemic. A small matter such as the distance between beds might have made a significant difference in infection rates within the hospitals.

By the end of the war, commodities price inflation was exacerbating hospital debts; hospital staples such as medicines, coal, grain, potatoes, sugar and alcohol had all increased in price. The influx of patients during the pandemic added an extra burden to their finances as well as their services. Cork Street's debt in March 1919 was £2,500. The Inspectors of Dublin Hospitals in their report for the epidemic year praised the hospital's performance with limited means during the epidemic, commenting that such an institution was vital to every city as it removed infectious diseases cases from the homes of the poor.[3] They begged that none of the 260 fever beds in the hospital be closed; the cost of each bed per patient, they argued, was about one third the cost of a bed in similar institutions in other cities. By the following year, the additional patient numbers Cork Street had treated in the influenza year had impacted on its finances. The debt had more than doubled to £5,882, in another busy year for the hospital as it dealt with the lingering effects of the influenza epidemic into April and May, and an outbreak of measles.

No comparative statistics on illness and death from individual disease are available for the Adelaide, a charitable Dublin hospital with a Protestant ethos and admission policy. Instead, the hospital's annual reports offer indications of the pressures that were probably common to all hospitals dealing with the unusually high numbers of influenza patients at a time when their finances were already so critical that they impinged on normal operations. The annual report for the year ending 31 December 1918 noted that in comparison to the pre-war standard, food had increased in price by 100 per cent, coal and light by 140 per cent, drugs and surgical appliances by 80 per cent; the expenditure under these headings rising from £4,205 in 1913 to £7,929 in 1918. The hospital had been forced to make two extra fundraising appeals in the autumn of 1918 as the influenza epidemic was at its zenith, one to regular subscribers and another, a 'half crown fund' to bring in smaller sums from former patients. At the end of the year the hospital had a bank overdraft of £4,062, and was under threat of closure if it could not increase its income or reduce its expenditure. From mid-summer, the financial crisis had forced hospital management to take economy measures that would later impinge on the influenza epidemic. They issued orders to ration heat on the wards: patients were to be kept for longer periods in bed during cold weather; fires could only be lit on wards at night by leave from matron; and surgeons were to operate on as few days as possible. Fires were banned in the bed-sitting rooms and dining room of the nurses' home; the house surgeon's fire was to be lit only when needed. It is perhaps a measure of the success of these economising schemes that at the height of the epidemic in November 1918 hospital management ordered that the coal cellar under the hospital's dispensary be locked.[4]

Many of the Adelaide's ten nursing sisters and forty-three nurses and probationers became ill during the autumn outbreak of influenza, when the wards were crowded with severe influenza and pneumonia cases. The hospital management committee expressed its thanks to those nursing staff who were able to remain on duty, and to Voluntary Aid Detachment (VAD) nurses who helped out: 'The year was characterized by two outbreaks of influenza. That in the autumn was very severe, a large number of the nursing staff were attacked, some very seriously, at a time when the wards were crowded with bad cases, especially of pneumonia. A very great strain was thrown on the members of the nursing staff who were able to remain on duty.'[5]

The Adelaide's medical report for 1918 reveals that 474 patients were admitted to the medical wards during the year. The pandemic of influenza caused a severe strain on the hospital accommodation. A reduction in the numbers of soldiers seeking admission enabled the staff to accommodate more influenza patients in the Victoria Home; otherwise even more hardship would have been inflicted on the sick poor. According to the medical officer, the increased death rate was entirely due to the serious nature of many of the pneumonia cases admitted, some of whom died only hours after admission to the hospital. The peak months for admission to the hospital in 1918 were June, and October, November and December, reflecting the first and second waves. The influenza pandemic continued to place pressure on the hospital and the staff in the first four months of 1919, according to the annual medical report compiled by Dr George Peacocke. Some 398 patients were admitted to the medical wards in 1919.[6] Dr Peacocke, physician to the Adelaide and the King George V hospitals in Dublin, claimed in November 1918 that there had been 497 influenza admissions during the month of October 'in a large hospital where he worked, to which milder cases were not admitted, with thirty-two deaths, a percentage of 6.5.'[7] Although he does not name the hospital, it might be assumed that he refers to the Adelaide which was rather bigger than the 110-bed King George V Military Hospital.

Some hospital records can be astonishingly silent on the crisis.[8] The records of Sir Patrick Dun's Hospital in Dublin, housed in the heritage centre at the Royal College of Physicians in Ireland, do not include any patient registers for the years in question; the minute books of meetings of medical staff contain nothing relevant; the Board of Governors' minute book's entire discussion of the pandemic is a minute of the board's condolences to the family of two nurses who died and a reference to a nurse who was allowed to complete her certificate early as nurses were required in the time of 'national emergency'; the most expansive references were in the post-mortem record book, and even there, in only two cases was the word influenza mentioned.[9]

By comparison, D.W. Macnamara's personal account of his experience working as a new house doctor in the Mater Misericordiae hospital in Dublin during the epidemic is an evocative description of what it was like to work on the ground in hospitals in Dublin during the crisis.[10]

The Mater normally had a couple of fever wards in operation, just sufficient, as Macnamara joked, for the medical authorities to be satisfied that young doctors would acquire a competent knowledge of fever. During the epidemic almost every ward in the house was transformed in to a fever ward, with just one gynaecological ward and one male and one female surgical ward retained for emergencies. He believed that the number of influenza patients he had examined must have 'run well into four figures'. He saw up to fifteen bodies in the mortuary at one time and six or seven were commonplace. He once examined a newly admitted case at 4 pm, and another in the same bed three hours later, as the previous patient had died and been removed to the mortuary.[11]

The National Archives in Kew holds documents submitted by the Irish command for the *Medical History of the War*. The report was sent to the editorial team in 1920 when the memory of influenza pandemic was still fresh, and indicates a clear understanding that a phenomenon out of the ordinary, even for exceptional times, had occurred. These records list the numbers admitted and deaths during the three waves of the epidemic to the King George V: 190 soldiers were admitted and sixteen died in July 1918, 768 admitted with seventy-eight dying on October and November 1918 which the author described as the most severe wave, and 411 were admitted with forty-four deaths in February and March 1918. The report said half the hospital staff were felled by the disease, and praised the staff for their 'excessive work under very trying conditions'. Hospital authorities filled whatever space they could with extra beds: 150 were added in huts, wards and a passage. Even as they struggled to cope with the epidemic forty-eight injured soldiers were brought in from the torpedoed *RMS Leinster* in October 1918; 175 bodies were also brought into the hospital, of which 143 being buried in the military cemetery in Grangegorman.[12] The Royal Navy did not have hospital accommodation in Lough Swilly and so their casualties were sent either to the military hospital or the county infirmary in Derry, which kept thirty beds for naval and military personnel during the war. Between 4,000 and 6,000 troops in the Ulster brigade area – which stretched from Athlone to Belfast – fell ill with flu in June and July 1918. Adopting 'strenuous hygiene measures ... to combat the epidemic ... brought out a great decline in the number of cases'. During the next outbreak from October 1918 to March 1919, 2,166 soldiers were diagnosed with influenzal illness. Patients were treated locally in camps or barracks, but immediately isolated. Anti-influenzal vaccine was administered in Finner camp, and troops were instructed on pain of punishment to allow air to move freely through the sleeping areas.

The Curragh military hospital in County Kildare had 230 cases described as 'broncho-pneumonia', with a mortality rate of 9 per cent during the epidemic. This rate of death was lower than in other military hospitals; the Curragh medical staff accredited the success to an atropine-based treatment method they had developed. Patients treated with vaccines did not do well, often developing secondary infections, so treatment was discontinued. Pfeiffer's bacillus grew regularly on the blood agar growth medium, but the army doctors were not convinced Pfeiffer's was the exclusive cause. Having tried creosote vaccines and many of the other treatments recommended in the literature, they used an initial hypodermic injection of atropine and digitalis to localise and limit the pulmonary infection. They understood a diffuse bronchitis as a 'wet condition of the lung [which] is conducive to spread of infection'. The atropine would dry or prevent the wetting of the lungs. If the lungs dried up the patient was kept comfortable and given plenty of fluids. If they were still wet, the staff would repeat the atropine or mix it with belladonna. A different presentation, the 'confluent' type, which had 'a toxic condition' on top of the severe pulmonary infection, and the patient was cyanosed was considered serious. 'The prognosis is always grave, but not so hopeless as one would believe from the literature. We have seen several recoveries from septic pneumonia, almost hopeless cases – pessimism is a bad physician.' They said the flu was widespread in the Curragh camp during the autumn of 1918, but that it did not seem to be as severe in the camp as in the surrounding towns. The Royal Army Medical Corps (RAMC) doctors went out to help the civilian doctors when they were overwhelmed with work, which suggests that the problem was greater in the civilian population.

Mental hospitals and institutions

Some 234 deaths in the district and auxiliary lunatic asylums were directly attributed to influenza in 1918. Pneumonia, bronchitis and pleurisy, all possible sequelae of influenza, accounted for another 236 deaths, giving a total of 470 deaths possibly caused by the epidemic out of a total of 2,243 deaths in the lunatic asylums in 1918. Almost 21 per cent of all deaths in the lunatic asylums could be attributed to the pandemic in 1918.[13] The situation improved slightly in 1919, perhaps because as a relatively closed group, some had acquired immunity in 1918. There were ninety-two deaths certified as influenza, while 148 died from pneumonia, bronchitis and pleurisy. The total number of deaths was 1,796, also down significantly on the previous year. One in seven died from influenza or related illnesses during the year, and the deaths represented just over 13 per cent of the total number of deaths in the asylums.[14] In their report for 1918, the inspectors note that the deaths in 1918 exceeded the deaths in 1917 by fifty-two, and that the general death rate per cent of the daily average number resident in the asylums was 11.1. The general death rate was only 0.6 per cent higher than in 1917; the inspectors note that in the previous year's report they had commented on the great increase in the death rate in 1917, which had been attributed to a combination of a prolonged cold spell accompanied by an outbreak of influenza, and the adverse effect of the war on the food and other supplies. 'As the same causes operated in 1918, a reduction in the heavy death rate could hardly be expected.'[15]

The highest death rate in any mental asylum during 1918 was in Belfast asylum, 19.7 per cent of the average resident number. Carlow asylum had an outbreak of influenza in October and November; its death rate for the year was above average, at 13.7 per cent of the average resident number. The death rate at Enniscorthy's asylum remained exactly the same as the previous year, at 11.9 per cent of the average resident number. Kilkenny reported cases of influenza throughout the year; the heaviest outbreak was in November and the death rate as a percentage of the average resident number rose to 14 per cent in 1918, from 8.1 per cent in 1917. Maryborough also had influenza throughout the year, with most in October and November, and the death rate rising to 14.2 per cent. Mullingar escaped lightly; its death rate was slightly below the general average for 1918 at 10.9 per cent. Dublin's Richmond asylum had two outbreaks of influenza, in July and in October–November. The other Dublin asylum, Portrane, also had outbreaks of influenza in early summer and in November. The death rate for the two asylums, grouped together by the inspectors, was extremely low, at 8.6 per cent of the average resident number. The Criminal Lunatic Asylum at Dundrum, Co. Dublin, had some cases of influenza from August, but no deaths were recorded. The inspectors also reported that influenza was listed as a principal cause or factor in the insanity of forty-six males and fifty-six female patients admitted to the asylums during the year, although they do not give any indications of what types of insanity it caused. Of the 234 deaths from influenza, fifty-four were below the age of thirty, out of a total 315 deaths in this age group. In the thirty–sixty age group, 142 people died from influenza; thirty-eight of the people who died from influenza were aged over sixty. These age groups are so broad they do not lend themselves to any meaningful analysis, but the general evidence demonstrates the benefits of isolation.

The prison service and the influenza epidemic

The Irish GPB claimed in official reports that only one prisoner died from influenza in Irish prisons during the entire epidemic period. That prisoner, a female inmate of Derry jail, died from influenza complicated by double pneumonia in October 1918. The GPB's report for the year 1918–19 stated that of the other three prisoners who died in local and convict prisons, two succumbed to bronchitis followed by heart failure, and another prisoner died from heart failure shortly after admission to prison; there remains a possibility that influenza may have had a bearing on these deaths. Ten prisoners suffering from influenza were granted an early release from Belfast jail in July 1918, November and December 1918, being sent either to hospital or home. One prisoner in Galway jail suffering from influenza, was released to hospital in November 1918. One prisoner in Mountjoy jail in Dublin, who was suffering from influenza and pneumonia, was released to Dr Steevens Hospital on 29 October 1918.[16]

The health of prisoners in Irish jails during the year 1919–20 was, according to the annual report of the GPB, remarkably good, with influenza being the only real health issue. Only four 'local' prisoners died in prison that year: three from heart failure and one from injuries caused by bullet wounds. No prisoners died in the convict prisons.[17] Four prisoners were released from Mountjoy jail because they were suffering from influenza between 12 March and 14 March 1919; on 12 March, a thirty-six-year-old male prisoner admitted on 18 February 1919 was released and sent to the South Dublin Union hospital, having developed influenza and pneumonia. A nineteen-year-old male prisoner, in jail since 21 March 1918, was sent to Cork Street Fever Hospital suffering from influenza and tachycardia (a faster than normal heartbeat) on the same date. The following day, 13 March 1919, a twenty-year-old male prisoner suffering from influenza, who had been imprisoned since 30 January 1919, was also released to Cork Street Hospital. On 14 March 1919, a twenty-three-year-old male prisoner, admitted to prison on 21 September 1918, was sent to the Mater Hospital with influenza. The fate of those prisoners released to hospital care while suffering from influenza is not documented in the reports in either year; it would seem likely that if prisoners with influenza were so ill that the prison authorities felt it expedient to release them, whether to hospital or to home, then they could not have been suffering from a mild case.[18] The prison authorities may have been motivated by something other than concern for the prisoner' health, particularly where political prisoners were involved. Sinn Féin had long been promoting the concept that political prisoners were mistreated by the Government. Releasing influenza victims before they succumbed to the illness would have meant that their deaths did not become a statistic for propaganda use.

There were some differences between the ways in which the three prisons boards – for Ireland, for Scotland and for England and Wales – officially reported the influence of influenza pandemic on prisons in the different jurisdictions. Six prisoners died from disease in Scottish prisons during the year 1918; only one of the six was attributed to influenza. In contrast to the Irish reports, the annual report of the Prison Commissioners for Scotland listed not only those who died in prison, but also those prisoners who died after being transferred on medical grounds to general hospitals. There were eleven of these deaths in 1918, of which three were from pneumonia. The Scottish commissioners also documented the numbers of prisoners suffering from influenza and related illnesses: there were 264 prisoners treated in jail for influenza, and all but one recovered. There were 281 cases of bronchitis, also a consequence or alternative diagnosis of influenza.[19] During 1919, there were two deaths from influenza in Scottish prisons, and two prisoners transferred to general hospitals on medical grounds died from pneumonia. The report notes that the death rate among prisoners, including those transferred to hospital, was 6 per thousand living, which the authorities considered remarkable in view of the fact that Scotland had experienced such a severe influenza epidemic during the year. Five prisoners were transferred to general hospitals because of influenza, ten because of pneumonia, and three due to bronchitis.[20] In England and Wales, there were fifty-one deaths from natural causes in local prisons in the year ending 31 March 1919. Forty-two of these were male and nine were female. In convict prisons, there were twenty-one deaths from natural causes, eighteen males and three females. In both types of prison, the death rate was far higher than in the previous year, and this is ascribed to the influenza epidemics. In local prisons there were fourteen influenza deaths, and in convict prisons there were thirteen deaths from influenza and influenzal pneumonia.[21] During the year ending 31 March 1920, the report of the commissioners of prisons for

England and Wales noted that there was a marked absence of influenza, and that the level of infectious disease generally continued to be very low, which, the report said, reflected the general satisfactory sanitary condition of the prisons. In the convict prisons, thirteen died, twelve males and one female; the death rate from natural causes per thousand of the daily average population was 7.9, as against 16.5 in 1918–19, with the difference between the two rates being attributed by the authorities to the influenza epidemics.[22]

The voluminous correspondence of Ireland's General Prisons Board suggests that influenza made a greater impression on the prisons service than the annual reports indicate. Throughout the epidemic period, sheaves of the correspondence refer to the influenza epidemic and the various effects it was having on Irish prisons. The correspondence also deals with the tensions over influenza among political prisoners and internees, which is explored in the next chapter. One significant theme that emerges is that the influenza impacted severely on prison warders on their families, whose healthcare was covered by the prisons' medical service. Aside from those situations, the letters are typically about shortages of staff through illness or to attend the funerals of family members who had succumbed to influenza. Several warders were granted compassionate leave to care for their families when their wives became ill. Warders were constantly being moved from prison to prison to replace staff ill with influenza. Influenzal attacks suffered by the families of prison staff placed an extra burden on the prison doctors, as they also provided treatment for prison staff and their families. Deaths of warders and members of their families were not unusual. Governor Munro of Mountjoy telephoned the GPB on 22 October 1918 on receipt of a wire from Warder Newman of Kilkenny prison asking for a warder to replace Chief Warder George Cullen, who was off-duty with influenza; Munro mentioned that fourteen of his officers were away owing to illness, leave of absence or temporary duty. Max Green, chairman of the GPB, sanctioned the sending of a warder for temporary duty to Kilkenny; Warder James Dillane was duly sent. In a letter dated the same day to the Governor of Mountjoy, Newman warned that as his own wife was ill with influenza, he expected to fall victim to it at any moment himself. In compliance with prison regulations, Warder Dillane reported to Governor Munro the two following days that the prison doctor had attended to Chief Warder Cullen and his family at their home in Prison Terrace. Cullen and three of his children, Ella, Jack and Alfred, were by then in bed, suffering from influenza. Another son, George, had pneumonia. Mrs Cullen and another son Charles were convalescent. On 26 October, Dillane forwarded to Munro Dr Brennan's report that Cullen's two sons Charles and John were convalescing, his son Alfred and daughter Ella were still suffering from influenza, and that his third son George had become seriously ill with pneumonia. The forty-four-year-old chief warder died from pneumonia on 28 October 1918.[23] Shortly after his death, his wife was informed that their eight-year-old son George had also died from the same disease, at the County Infirmary.[24] Mr Cullen's legal representatives were given a gratuity of £123 15s 8d under the terms of the Superannuation Act, 1909; the award was later increased, although no details of the revised award were revealed.

Warder Newman's family seemed to recover from influenza, with his wife and two children having been treated by Dr James.[25] The warder sent from Mountjoy to replace the chief warder, James Dillane, lost his thirty-year-old wife Mary Theresa Dillane to septic pneumonia, following influenza, on 23 March 1919.[26] Although Cullen's family received some financial compensation for his death, sudden death from influenza caused unexpected financial hardship for the surviving families of warders who had not accepted the 1909 pension scheme – an issue revealed by a series of correspondence about Warder Patrick Irwin of Mountjoy, who died on 15 November from influenzal pneumonia. Irwin had joined the prison service aged twenty-two in 1903; he had no insurance and no pension. His colleagues wrote to the GPB, asking for financial assistance for his widow, as she had no money to pay the funeral expenses and none of her friends were in a position to help financially. The couple had four small children. Max Green replied as follows on behalf of the board: 'The board much regret that they have no funds at their disposal which could be applied in this case.'[27] As senior warders with families were usually provided with accommodation as part of their terms and conditions of employment, the death of a warder meant not only the tragic loss of a family member and the possible loss of the sole source of family income, but also the loss of the family home.[28]

The reports of influenza illness among the prison population were peppered with cautious notes stating that in the case of prisoners ill with influenza, every proper action had been taken. This was particularly evident in the correspondence about the only recognised death of a prisoner in an Irish jail from influenza – the female prisoner in Derry jail in October 1918. The young married woman, aged twenty-four, a native of Fintona, died in prison on 20 October. She had been out on bail for trial at the Omagh sessions on 16 October for larceny of a clock and a gold watch, and after conviction was committed to the prison. She was seen by the medical officer on the next day and appeared in good health. On 18 October, when she complained about feeling ill, the medical officer placed her under medical treatment. The medical officer, in consultation with another doctor, examined her carefully and came to the conclusion that she had double pneumonia; they tried to get a nurse, as they considered her condition critical, and in the meantime an assistant matron was nursing her around the clock. They saw her again on the morning of 20 October, and noted that there was a marked tendency to heart failure, with very little air passing into the lungs. At 2.45 pm the doctor received a call from the governor to say that she was much worse; by the time they arrived at 2.57 pm the prisoner was dead. She had been seen twice by the chaplain before her death. The coroner's jury report from 21 October found that the prisoner had died from influenza complicated by double pneumonia and heart failure.[29]

The coal shortage severely affected the prisons during the epidemic and placed further obstacles in the way of prison staff endeavouring to care for influenza sufferers. The GPB had sent a memorandum to the prisons during the peak weeks of the epidemic in the autumn of 1918 requesting them to concentrate the prisoners in certain areas and to do anything else in their power to reduce the number of fires in furnaces and grates, and not to use gas lights unnecessarily.[30]

Correspondence between Mountjoy prison officials and the GPB intensified in March 1919 when there was an outbreak of the disease in the prison during the third wave of the epidemic. Probably keenly aware of both the trouble influenza had caused among the prisoners in Belfast and of the negative publicity from the contemporaneous outbreak of influenza among the 'German' plot internees in Gloucester jail, the prison authorities kept an anxious watch for a few days on the Mountjoy influenza situation.[31] The Mountjoy medical officer noted in his journal on 6 March 1919, the day that 'German' plot internee Pierce McCan died from influenza in Gloucester, that he had made arrangements for the disinfection of all cells from which prisoners had been removed suffering from influenza; forwarding this note to the GPB Governor Munro added: 'There are fresh cases this evening.'[32] There followed a series of correspondence between the board and officials at Mountjoy, usually Governor Munro, reporting daily on the health of prisoners suffering from influenza, and what measures the prison medical staff were taking to treat the prisoners and to prevent the spread of the disease. On 7 March 1919, the medical officer reported that there were eight new cases in the male prison hospital, and that if the epidemic spread more there would be a difficulty isolating the patients, although every precaution was being taken to prevent that happening.[33] On 8 March 1919, Munro submitted an extract from the medical officer's journal to the chairman of the board, Max Green, reporting that the influenza patients were progressing satisfactorily so far, and that there were two fresh cases that day.[34] The General Prisons' Board (GPB) was so interested in the influenza situation in Mountjoy that its medical member, Dr MacCormack, visited the Mountjoy prison on 9 March to see the conditions himself.

Clonmel Borstal helping the community

When more than 2,000 people in Clonmel, Co. Tipperary became ill in November 1918, the town's doctors asked Governor Dobbin of Clonmel Borstal and the Red Cross for urgent help. Governor Dobbin wrote to the GPB to inform them that he and his staff were assisting, as there had been many deaths among the poorer families 'for want of nourishment and fuel'. The borstal provided hot Bovril and soups for the most pressing cases, boiling the water in the institution's cookhouse and delivering fifteen gallons of hot soup each day with the help of Red Cross ladies. Other ladies with pony traps drove around the town and outskirts serving out the soup to the needy poor, many of whom were bedridden. When the town corporation took over with the help of donations from the public, the borstal handed over a list of about a hundred houses requiring help. Dobbin stated: 'There can be no doubt that prompt action has saved the lives of several who had neither food nor coal or the ability to wait upon themselves.' The officer in charge of the cookhouse and several of the inmates helped to prepare the huge quantities of soup without, he claimed, interfering with the usual work or incurring any costs. Dobbin said that the borstal took every precaution to prevent the epidemic entering the institution itself, and asked that the Board to approve the institution's efforts to help the ill in the community, which they did. Dobbin also requested a supply of vaccine for the boys and the institution's staff and their families. Dr McCormack of the Prisons Board rejected this request on two grounds: that the consent of the boys or their parents would have to be obtained before they were vaccinated, and that he did not consider vaccination to be effective.

Despite Sinn Féin's protestations to the contrary – statistics suggest that during the influenza epidemic prison was a relatively safe place to be, provided one was a prisoner. For warders and their families, who were less socially isolated than the prisoners, the picture was rather different, as both the GPB correspondence and the RG's statistics indicate.

Collectively, the correspondence on the pandemic's effects on the prison service shows the strong communication channels between prisons and the board.

Schools and colleges

What of influenza in schools? As we saw in Chapter 2, they were frequently closed for long periods during the epidemic, and that there was an understanding that children were somehow more likely to pass the disease on than other age groups. And yet the relevant annual report of the Irish Commissioners of National Education is disappointingly reticent about the effects of the disease on pupils and teachers. The commissioners noted that average daily attendance at national schools was the lowest for several years, dropping to 68.9 per cent of those on the rolls owing to the outbreak in the autumn and winter of 1918, but improving somewhat in 1919.[35] This is the only mention in the entire report of the disease; they mention the number of teachers who died during the year, but not the causes. We know from other sources cited in this work that some teachers died from this influenza, and we also know that people whose work involved dealing with the public, like the police, medical doctors and nurses, shop workers and bank staff died in greater numbers than those who worked in more isolated ways, so it would seem probable that many teachers also died during the pandemic.

THE LOWER LINE 327

Oct. 20th—More and more poor sick fellows with the " flu " are going in every day, and after every meal there is a rush to that part of the infirmary where you are weighed in the balance and usually found wanting in a sufficiency of temperature (excuse the expression)

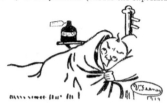

which is necessary to get you to bed. More excitement. The " flu " has gained a firm grip on Clongowes. The gymnasium is reported to be almost full, and plans are on foot to turn the III. Line top dormitory into a ward. At present we have four nurses.

Oct. 22nd—The games are just now completely disorganised, for there are so few in each Division that all the Divisions have to be amalgamated. The result is a very scrappy sort of match. In Rugby it seems to be nothing but scrums, for the uncivilised former members of 2nd and 3rd Divisions seem to have a strange passion for throwing the ball forward, and such little details as off-side are unknown or ignored completely by them.

Oct. 28th—Only the really hardy members of the house are now outside the infirmary walls—*i e.*, the lower infirmary, the "top" infirmary, the gym, the III. Line top dormitory, and, finally, even a part of the Lower Line dormitory. Everything seems upset, classes are amalgamated or changed, for the Community have not escaped unscathed.

Nov. 2—We were all very sorry and very surprised when Father Rector announced this morning the death of one of our schoolfellows, poor **Willie Carroll**. He was a very quiet sort of boy, so that he was not very well known to all, but some of us who happened to become more intimate with him knew him to be pious, truly generous, and " decent," as we call it, in every sense of the word, and, of course, his cleverness was known to all, a genius that would have brought him glory at school and success when he left us.

Nov. 5th—Father Minister solemnly announced the fact, amid " loud cheers and laughter," that owing to very great pressure of work on the laundry people during the " flu," we should have to make our own beds in the morning. Strange to say, I noticed several taking down their rugs from the study to the dormitory, presumably to keep them warm, and yet if one contracts a habit of being one of the last out of the dormitory it is so very easy to slip a rug over a half-made bed ; but, of course, I don't make any insinuations.

Nov. 7th—Fr. Rector very kindly gave us one hour's pictures to-night. Charlie Chaplin in " A Dog's Life" reduced the audience to fits of laughter.

Nov. 12th—To-day is a playday in honour of **St. Stanislaus**, and, sad to say, to-day ends the free time we have had for more than a week. This evening, too, the Rector very kindly showed us a very good film on the **cinema**, which he only procured after great trouble, called " The Honour System," connected with American prison life. To-day was concluded our Chess Tournament, which ended in a victory for Allen O'Meara, who played a fine solid game all through. It was a very great success, and evidently some are great adepts at the game.

Nov. 24th—This evening the Lower Line **Debating Society** held its first meeting and the speeches were excellent, much better than had been anticipated, as the subject, " Polar Exploration," was rather a difficult one.

Dec. 1st—To-day were played the Inter-Line **Cup Matches**, and we Lower Liners pitted a great many teams against the Higher Line and the III. Line. The result was not quite so satisfactory perhaps as we had hoped, but the games, owing to the " flu," have been completely disorganised for some time past. However, our First Division XI. made a drawing with a very strong team from II. Division Higher Line, and led by Billy Lyons played a very good game, our aforementioned Captain particularly distinguishing himself.

Dec. 2nd—This evening we were entertained by a splendid **Concert**, to which the whole Line was admitted, and we had an enjoyable evening listening to the musical strains of the L L. Choral Society and the solos of Jack Delaney and Joe O'Dwyer, but the most novel item of the evening was afforded by Jack O'Mahony, who danced the Sailor's Hornpipe, and was magnificently arrayed in white ducks and a complete sailor's rig-out. Our especial thanks are due to Mr. Croasdaile, whose unwearied labours had their fruit in the splendid choruses sung this evening. Here is our programme :—

G

Figure 14 An extract from the *Clongownian* on how the disease interrupted school life, 1919.

As in the case of the hospitals, the quality and quantity of information that archives of schools and universities offer about the pandemic vary. Some, like those of Trinity College, Dublin, seem not to have recorded it, even though Professor R.B. McDowell recalled that hearing Botany Bay Square was used as a makeshift centre for students suffering from the disease (Chapter 7). Others reveal much about the pandemic and how it was managed within, particularly if some form of personal account or diary exists.

The minister of Clongowes Wood College in rural Co. Kildare, Fr Potter, kept a daily journal describing vividly the epidemic's effects on staff and pupils, and how the school managed it. The Irish Catholic élite's equivalent of Eton, Clongowes Wood had a hundred-year-long tradition of educating politicians, medical doctors, lawyers and soldiers (one of the pupils in the autumn of 1918 was James Deeney, who would later revolutionise Irish public health, as the government's chief medical adviser).[36] Both Fr Potter's journal and the college's annual journal the *Clongownian* permit the piecing together of an interesting picture of how the disease disrupted school life, and how management struggled to cope with it, using good nursing and social distancing to mitigate the effects of the disease.[37]

The flu entered Clongowes in mid-October, about the same time the epidemic's second and most severe of three waves was reaching its peak in the capital city. On the 16 October, the Rector awarded the pupils a 'playday', as the pupil numbers had reached a peak of 300 for the first time. The school celebrated with the showing of a film, 'A Man for All That', a black and white silent movie starring Elmer Clifton as a young convict. From entries in the minister's journal, it appears that film shows were a constant feature of college life at the time.

Three days later, on 19 October 1918, Fr Potter noted the first appearance of the epidemic: 'Influenza epidemic: Gymnasium turned into a ward. Three nurses from Town [Dublin]. Another nurse from town, and yet another.' An entry in the *Clongownian*, the school's annual journal notes: 'day by day, our ranks grow thinner. No longer is the question posed "How many have the Flu?", but instead, the question is "How many do not have the Flu?"', and that everyone was doing their best to avoid it. From another entry in the journal, it appeared that four or five days' starvation was part of the treatment.

By 23 October, the Minister wrote that ninety boys were 'down with the new influenza, a record in epidemics as far as CWC is concerned and more to come apparently'. College life was quite disrupted. The infirmary, top and bottom, the gym, the III Line top dormitory and even part of the lower dormitory were used to house the ill. Classes were amalgamated or changed, as the teaching staff was also affected. The disease spread like wildfire throughout the college: by the following day, it had felled 173 boys, nineteen servants, three nurses, five masters, one lay brother, the doctor, and four tradesmen, a total of 207; eleven nurses had been hired to care for them. By evening, the total number was 220. During the week, the school management changed the times of meals, probably in a desperate attempt to keep those not yet infected well. Influenza patients who were well enough to be eating were to have breakfast at 9 am, lunch at noon, dinner at 3.15 pm and tea at 7.30 pm; those who were not ill had their meals about half an hour earlier, probably to evade infection. Extra 'sleeps' were also ordered for the convalescent. Staff were advised not to attend the funerals of local people who had died from the disease, in another attempt to prevent further infection. With staff members being caught between a bind to comply with their employers' wishes, and a desire to pay respect to dead neighbours, funerals were arranged for after dark.

Disaster struck on 2 November, when a pupil, Willie Carroll died, from septic pneumonia, a frequent complication. His father had spent the last few days at his son's bedside. Again, probably in an attempt to limit the dangers of infection, no one was allowed into the room where he died for some time after. Requiem mass was held for him on 4 November. It was thought safer not to bring the corpse into the chapel. People who had recently had influenza were not allowed to enter the chapel and attend the funeral.

The deaths of two other pupils were also linked with influenza. Fr Potter described the death of George Lidwell as 'most mysterious'. Lidwell had complained of a sore shoulder a couple of days before Christmas Day, an injury that was initially believed from a fall into a pool of water and neglect to change his clothes. He was sent to the infirmary, where he had a temperature of 101 on admission, which crept up to 107 degrees Fahrenheit over the next few days. The college doctor and a consultant from 'town' (Dublin) were called in to treat him as his condition worsened. His mother and sister and brother came to stay at his bedside. He died on 26 December. His body was taken up to Gardiner St on the afternoon of the 27 December for the funeral the following day, which was attended by the rector and three scholastics. The minister noted in his diary that the possible diagnoses for the mysterious death included acute rheumatism, osteomyelitis and influenza. The third boy to die, Donal Gorman, had been one of those who had fallen ill with influenza in October. He was still ailing after the initial attack had passed, and was taken home to Dublin; the school community learned of his death in January. A marble tablet was erected to the memory of all three boys by their fellow students, which is still visible at the college chapel door.

The pages of the *Clongownian* marked the deaths of several past pupils who died from the disease. Included in their number was Pierce McCan, the charismatic Tipperary farmer and nationalist, who died while interned in Gloucester for alleged involvement in the 'German' plot – trumped up charges against prominent nationalists and anti-conscription campaigners in the run-up to the pivotal 1918 general election (see Chapter 8).

Clongowes Wood management, in their practice of social distancing, the hiring of extra nursing staff, and the provision of extra food and rest for the convalescent, were clearly following the best contemporary medical advice. Given that this strain of influenza killed an average of 2.5 per cent of those infected, together with the fact that only three died out of 220 ill pupils, indicates that the disease management and treatment policy within the college was reasonably successful.

In St Patrick's College, Maynooth, there was a severe outbreak during both the second and third waves of the epidemic, in the winter of 1918 and the spring of 1919. The college president's annual report for 1918–19 also shows that the authorities there also tried to limit the outbreak through social distancing:

> At first it was hoped that by carefully isolating the patients and by suspending classes for a while it might be possible to prevent it from spreading, but all these measures proved ineffectual. The situation was rendered still more alarming by the fact that nearly all the domestics were stricken down, and no extra nursing help could be procured. Sir Joseph Redmond, MD, the consulting physician, was invited to visit the college and to advise what should be done. At the conference held to discuss the

matter it was fully recognised by all parties that, whether the students were retained or sent away, the risks were great, but as there were few servants and as no nurses could be procured, it was decided as the lesser of two evils to close the college. When this decision was announced to the students, an appeal was made to them that no one who felt unwell should leave the college without the permission of the doctor.

Sixty students were retained as patients in the Infirmaries, and the remainder left the college on the 8th November. Thanks to the skill and attention of the Sisters of Charity and the doctor, there were no deaths in the college either among the students or the domestics. But, unfortunately, the same cannot be said of those who went home. Eleven students died from the effects of influenza.[38]

In February, the disease broke out in St Patrick's once more. Within a few days, about 160 students and several members of the administrative and teaching staff were affected. When the infirmaries were filled to overflowing, the class halls in the Junior House were turned into temporary hospital wards.

Looking back over this chapter on what institution records tell us about the influenza crisis, we see a wide variety in the types of information that institutional records offer on this sometimes crucial episode in their history. From rich archives like those of the prison service or Clongowes Wood College we can piece together different sources to create a passable narrative of just how the influenza impinged on the daily life of people within in these institutions, and how their management reacted to reduce the impact on their institution. Annual reports like those of the hospitals can also give a different sort of window into the 1918 influenza story, showing the financial problems it provoked or worsened.

Notes

1 Medical report for The House of Recovery and Fever Hospital, Cork St Dublin the for the year ending 31 March 1920. RCPI heritage centre.
2 Medical report for the House of Recovery and Fever Hospital, Cork St Dublin the for the year ending 31 March 1920. RCPI heritage centre.

3 Sixty-first annual report of the Board of Superintendence of the Dublin Hospitals for the year 1918–1919, cmd 480.

4 Sixty-first annual report of the Adelaide and Fetherston-Haugh convalescent home, Rathfarnham, for 1918, Adelaide Archive, Trinity College, Dublin. Adelaide Hospital finance and house committee minutes, 1918.

5 Sixty-first annual report of the Adelaide and Fetherston-Haugh convalescent home, Rathfarnham, for 1918, Adelaide Archive, Trinity College, Dublin.

6 Medical reports of the Adelaide Hospital for 1918 and 1919, Adelaide Archive, Trinity College, Dublin.

7 *The Medical Press*, 1 January 1919.

8 The Survey of Hospital Archives in Ireland 2015 report by the National Archives of Ireland funded by the Wellcome Trust described surviving historic hospital and healthcare records as 'generally vulnerable' and in need of clear guidelines on research access.

9 Post-mortem book, 27 February 1919, Sir Patrick Dun's hospital archive, Royal College of Physicians in Ireland Heritage Centre.

10 Macnamara, 'Memories of 1918 and "the Flu"', p. 304.

11 Macnamara, 'Memories of 1918 and "the Flu"'.

12 National Archives: WO35/1794. Call for historical review of medical work in the Irish command during the war period. The information was collated for inclusion in the *Medical History of the War*.

13 *The sixty-eighth annual report (with appendices) of the Inspectors of Lunatics, for the year ending 31 December 1918* (1920), xxi, cmd 579.

14 *The sixty-ninth annual report (with appendices) of the Inspectors of Lunatics (Ireland) for the year ending 31 December 1919* (1921), xv, cmd 1127.

15 *The sixty-eighth annual report (with appendices) of the Inspectors of Lunatics.*

16 *Forty-first report of the General Prisons Board, Ireland, 1918–1919* (1920), xxiii, cmd 687.

17 *Forty-second report of the General Prisons Board, Ireland, 1919–1920* (1921), xvi, cmd 13.

18 Ibid.

19 *Annual report of the Prison Commissioners for Scotland, for the year 1918* (1919), xxvii, cmd 78.

20 *Annual report of the Prison Commissioners for Scotland, for the year 1919* (1920), xxxiii, cmd 698.

21 *Report of the Commissioners of Prisons and the directors of convict prisons for 1918–1919* (1919), xxxvii, cmd 374.

22 *Report of the Commissioners of Prisons and the directors of convict prisons, 1919–20* (1920), xxiii, cmd 972.

23 General prisons board correspondence (GPB), 1918/6770; see also George Cullen's death registration at https://civilrecords.irishgenealogy. ie/churchrecords/images/deaths_returns/deaths_1918/05169/4426383. pdf (accessed 9 January 2017).

24 *Kilkenny People*, 2 November 1918; see also George Cullen's death registration at https://civilrecords.irishgenealogy.ie/churchrecords/images/deaths_ returns/deaths_1918/05169/4426383.pdf.

25 GPB, 1918/7097.

26 GPB, 1919/2375. See also Mary Theresa Dillane's death registration at https://civilrecords.irishgenealogy.ie/churchrecords/images/deaths_ returns/deaths_1919/05152/4420370.pdf (accessed 9 January 2017).

27 GPB, 1918/7463.

28 GPB, 1918/6996; 1918/ 6484.

29 GPB, 1918/6595.

30 GPB, 1918/6412.

31 Both of these issues will be discussed in Chapter 8.

32 GPB, 1919/1924.

33 GPB, 1919/1951.

34 GPB, 1919/1977.

35 *Eighty-fifth report of the commissioners of national education in Ireland, 1918–19*(cmd.1048) 1920.

36 For more on Deeny's substantial influence on Irish health, see Lawrence William White, Diarmaid Ferriter, 'Deeny, James Andrew', in James McGuire, James Quinn, eds, *Dictionary of Irish Biography.* (Cambridge: Cambridge University Press, 2009). (Available at http:// dib.cambridge.org/viewReadPage.do?articleId=a2499)

37 My thanks to the college's archivist, Margaret Doyle, for allowing me generous access to back issues of *The Clongownian,* the school's annual journal, and to the Minister's Journal.; also to Declan O'Keeffe, editor of *The Clongownian,* for directing me to the Clongowes archive.

38 Annual report of the President of St Patrick's College, Maynooth, 1918–19.

7

Dying and surviving: eye witnesses

Tommy Christian was a small boy of five when he woke in the middle of the night with a terrible pain in his throat; ninety-two years later he said 'you would never forget it'. He spoke of the dispensary doctor coming in his car – an 'old jalopy' – to treat his family, who were all ill with influenza, at three in the morning. His memories were so acute that the listener could hear the car pulling out outside the family home in north Kildare. Tommy did not realise at the time that he was part of the biggest disease event ever. Towards the end of his life, he was able, through the interview process, to make sense of what had happened to him and to his family. He and I came to see their intimate suffering and struggle to survive this illness as part of this much bigger national and global story of tragedy, of perhaps 50 million dead and half the world ill. He was, in a way, one of the lucky ones who lived to tell the tale; he died aged ninety-nine. However, his survival story was also tempered by tragedy.

This chapter draws on a collection of interviews with elderly child survivors of the pandemic, discussing their experiences after ninety years, and with members of families who had suffered a loss. When I began researching the subject in 2006 for my PhD in Trinity College Dublin, my supervisor Professor David Dickson convinced me that there was still a narrow window to collect living memory; he even provided the first interviewee. This was the historian and renowned TCD eccentric R.B. McDowell, who even in high summer could be seen walking around campus in an overcoat and woollen scarf. He caught it as a small boy in Belfast. These interviews show that the epidemic made a lasting impact on the memories of children, even though the event was puzzling as they did not have enough information to make sense of what was happening. They somehow knew it was important, perhaps internalising the anxious body language of the grown-ups fretting over them. Some became curious listeners, trying to glean scraps of information about it from newspapers and from hushed adult conversations.

Some had acute memories like Tommy's. For others, including R.B., the memory was hazy, mediated through a lens of febrile fog, the shadows of people moving around them, tending and anxiously hovering. Other interviewees told of family and neighbours who succumbed, sometimes leaving their loved ones to cope with not only emotional loss, but changed economic circumstances as well if the family breadwinner died; the loss of home and the separation of children are common findings. These stories not only tell of individual or familial trauma: but also they show how the medical system worked, the treatments that were given, the living conditions at the time and, most significantly, they add the human voice to impersonal records like death statistics and news reports.

Historians drawing together sources for looking at influenza in other geographic regions have made extensive use of memories of the disease. Two key oral histories of the pandemic have come from the southern hemisphere: Geoffrey Rice's *Black November: The 1918 Influenza Pandemic in New Zealand*, which first appeared in 1988, and Howard Phillip's *Black October. The Impact of the Spanish Influenza Epidemic of 1918 on South Africa*, which was published in 1990. Most notably, Richard Collier collected 1,708 individual accounts from people who had lived through the epidemic, in the form of letters, written accounts and interviews, publishing a selected few in his 1974 book *The plague of the Spanish Lady*. Collier did not interpret the interviews, but rather let them speak for themselves. He named each contributor and where they came from in an appendix; none were from Ireland. His collection was deposited with the Imperial War Museum in London.[1] Mark Honigsbaum used this collection as the primary source for his 2009 publication, *Living with Enza*; he interrogated some of Collier's interviews with Britons (Collier's subjects came from diverse global regions) and combined them with other material to capture the everyday experience of the disease in Britain.[2] Niall Johnson's *Britain and the 1918–19 Influenza Pandemic: a Dark Epilogue* drew extensively on references to the influenza in memoirs and biographies. Johnson has pointed to a conundrum that is a common feature about the recollection or documenting of individual experience of Spanish influenza in many geographic regions: while the epidemic left little trace on the collective memory, it often lingered beneath the surface in family histories:

> Here we have one of the three most devastating epidemics in history, and it occurred within living memory (just) and what do we have to show for it? In the local and national histories, in the national archives and in our collective memory, it has slipped away, leaving the merest of traces. Yet if we start to scratch the surface of our own family histories, we often find it.[3]

The US Government's Centers for Disease Control and Prevention (CDC) developed the *Pandemic Influenza Storybook* as a resource tool for public health professionals involved in a national programme on crisis and emergency risk communication. The online story book contains narratives from survivors, families and friends who lived through the 1918 and 1957 pandemics. CDC Director Dr Julie Gerberding has pointed out that collecting interviews with survivors of an influenza pandemic is about more than just recording history for the Centers:

> The stories on the website told so eloquently by survivors, family members, and friends from past pandemics, serve as a sobering reminder of the devastating impact that influenza can have and reading them is a must for anyone involved in public health preparedness.

These oral testimonies or memoirs enable us to develop insights into the effects of the disease which cannot be acquired from other sources. It is possible to acquire evidence about the social impact of the disease, how it affected individuals, families and communities in the short and long terms, and how it is perceived or construed by ordinary people, rather than in the less emotive terms of newspaper record or official documents and institutional records. Charles Rosenberg has shown that epidemic disease enables a cross-sectional view of cultural assumptions and responses. Robert A. Aronowitz has argued that the study of the effects of a disease on society is a useful exercise for the historian as disease can often evoke and reflect collective responses, so their study can provide an understanding of the values and attitudes of the society in which they occur. The Spanish influenza pandemic is a disease which is replete with social meaning.

In an international context that social meaning is loaded by its association with the First World War, while in an Irish context that association is further complicated by the association with key incidents in
the revolutionary period. There were political tensions over governance and public attitude towards the key organs of state, in particular
the LGB, which bore responsibility for public health. This was essentially exercised through its management of the Poor Law medical
dispensary system, which covered about 70 per cent of the Irish population. Influenza was, at once, one more trauma provided by the world
war experience, and something that cast a magnifying glass over the
British Government's arguably key interaction with the people, the
provision of healthcare and welfare by the LGB. Interviewing people
about the impact of the pandemic on individuals or small groups
could provide the opportunity not only to learn about the disease, but
also to obtain a bottom-up perspective on some of the key tensions in
Ireland of the 1910s.

Collecting influenza memories in Ireland

After a promising start with the McDowell interview, I started
searching for people who were old enough to have lived through it.
The challenge was to find reliable witnesses who would be willing
to be interviewed, trusting a stranger with intimate details of their
illness, their family circumstances and perhaps trauma. Some were
found by making contacts in nursing homes, through interviews
on the regional and national radio and articles in the regional and
national newspapers and in publications aimed specifically at the elderly. Eventually, as the project become better known, and as news
stories about the threats posed by avian and the 2009 H1N1 Influenza
A or 'Mexican' flu stimulated interest in and memory of this last
great influenza pandemic, people volunteered to participate. Some
participated in formal digitally recorded interviews; others, sometimes because of reticence, distance, or because they had not much
to impart, were interviewed by telephone or through written communication. In all, there are approximately fifty interviewees (some
scarcely count as interviews, being little more than a useful sentence,
whereas others contributed hours of recordings). I am indebted to
them all: their trust and their contributions provided a rewarding new
resource for the study of the pandemic.

The methods of the oral historian are complex; one has to learn interviewing techniques, to read people, to listen with care and to interpret silences. Joanna Bornat has written of the need for the interviewer to understand the effect that the interview has on the interviewee. When interviewing about a traumatic episode, the remembering can produce emotions that are difficult for both the interviewee and the interviewer to handle. Difficult, heavily considered passages of speech, long silences, and outbursts of long-forgotten emotion are commonplace. Some interviewees suggested that exploring the subject was in some way cathartic, enabling them to make sense of an event which they had previously seen as an isolated event of their childhood, and allowing them to place it within the context of the pandemic and a wider catastrophe. Rosenberg has argued that most people seek a rational understanding of threatening epidemics to minimise their sense of vulnerability; some of these interviewees had spent ninety years before being able to conceptualise their personal experience of Spanish flu in the wider framework of the disease.[4]

All researchers using oral history as a method face a set of concerns peculiar to their own work as well as the issues common to all. In the case of oral histories of Spanish influenza, there are particular issues about age and memory. The subjects who had direct experience of the pandemic were born before 1918; the youngest interviewee was born in 1915, the oldest in 1903. Even without taking into account their current physiological condition or the possibility of age-related brain degeneration, they were being asked to retrieve a memory that occurred ninety years earlier when they were small children with underdeveloped language, deductive or analytical skills. Dealing with people in their nineties and hundreds requires careful handling and some intuitive work. The researcher may have to revert to the social mores of a different era to obtain the best results, reassuring them that they are respected. For example, an introduction through a third party usually helps to set them at ease; and they often prefer to be given the option of being addressed formally. Elderly people often feel vulnerable, and the interviewer ought to be sensitive to their fears – foremost of which, usually, is that they are losing their memory. Some required reassurance that they might not remember the 'black flu' because it was outside their realm of experience; it might not have happened in their area, or have been spoken about in front of children. Often it proved possible to reassure them by asking them to retrieve another memory from this busy historic period. Most of the living witnesses did remember two other key events: the sinking of the *RMS Leinster* mail boat by a German torpedo in Dublin Bay in October 1918 when the flu was at its peak in Dublin, or the celebrations for the end of the war. Many also remembered personal experiences of the 1916 rebellion or the world war.[5]

The validity of the information offered by interviewees was checked against other sources, with the dual purpose of checking the authenticity of the evidence as well as discreetly checking the reliability of the individual's memory. Where there were noticeable but small errors, the errors have been corrected and noted. These, for the most part, concerned small likely errors of timing; the interviewee could refer to events taking place at a certain time, whereas from other sources it would seem the timing was incorrect. Some interviewees conflated the tuberculosis pandemic – the long epidemic – with the influenza pandemic. In this way, precautions were taken to support what Trevor Lummis stresses to be the main concern for oral history, the degree to which accurate recall of the past is possible.[6]

The interviews

R.B. McDowell, former Junior Dean at Trinity College, Dublin, spoke of his own experience of the illness. He came from a properous Belfast family, and at that stage he and his brother each had a nurse or nanny. He was five years of age, and remembered falling ill in October 1918; the doctor was called and told his family that the little boy was unlikely to last through the night. He survived, but could not recall what happened during his illness for the next three weeks or so.[7]

> I think I was unconscious, or delirious. I know I was very bad. I remember very little concrete, clearly … for the next ten years or more I recall the doctor being mildly irritated with me, as he had broken the news to my parents, in a very kind way, that I was not going to last the night. I think he thought I had acted in a revolutionary way, that I had defied the rules of medicine. Good nursing I heard was the only real remedy. Keeping warm and getting lots of warm drinks. I was lucky, I had good nursing. I was not conscious so I can't remember what I was given. Our household went down early. My parents had mild flu. It must have been mild flu. My father got up to celebrate

Armistice Day and went down town, the doctors disapproved of that, but I don't think he could have done that if it was not mild flu.

His brother's nurse (he suggested the term 'nanny' would be more appropriate now) died from influenza. The family doctor had managed to secure the McDowell family the services of a private nurse, at a time when there was an acute shortage of nurses; she took care of the young McDowell. The nurse lifted him to the window to hear the celebrations for the end of the war. He was considered sickly for a long time after having the flu, well into his teens, and was inclined to play that card to his own advantage for some years afterwards. Into his teens he was regarded as a delicate child, which he said had a 'mixed effect' on his character.

> It probably had the effect of weakening my resolution for hard work, you could always plead bad health. I was able up to the age of 12 or 14 to claim that I was an invalid, if school was too boring I could stay away; I think I expected a fair amount of indulgence, and could always get my own way, which inspires confidence. For years I could play the card of ill health. It certainly … I probably had at the back of my mind that the army was out, because of bad health, and, should I go to the bar, could I put up with the strain of being a barrister?

He recalled hearing 'grim stories' about the influenza. He told one story where a young soldier and his wife were found dead in their flat from flu, the alarm being raised by the crying of their baby; people broke into their flat to rescue the baby, and found the young couple dead. McDowell said there were many stories of that nature about the flu. A colleague at Trinity once told him that during the pandemic he came across an undergraduate who was suffering from the Spanish flu collapsed on the steps at the Exam Hall; the student was carried to Botany Bay, where there was a number of other undergraduates stretched out on the floor, waiting for ambulances. The attacks came on in hours, so people could be well leaving home in the morning, and seriously ill a few hours later. Asked where he thought the flu emerged from, he became a little and even uncharacteristically hesitant, as he pondered the issue.

> I think there was a vague belief that it was tied up with the war. There were grim stories coming from France that many people were down, in the army. It made a bigger impression on me than any other incident

since. I think, and this is a little speculative, that there was a kind of feeling, that people felt that having got through the war, it was unfair that the flu should strike. People felt that really it was unbelievable that people were dying who had got through the war, and had suffered from rationing. Flu made a tremendous impression, I think the only parallel would be the Black Death. For the later epidemics, there were better remedies, they seemed to have at least one remedy for later epidemics, so at least it was a fairer fight. Here, I think the defencelessness was a factor.

McDowell offered the opinion that most middle-class households would have had a maid, and would have easy access to doctors and possibly been able to acquire a private nurse, so good home nursing was possible and access to hospital was not a priority. He suggested that even for those in less fortunate circumstances hospitals did not have the same priority as they would now, that good home nursing by family or others was the key to recovering from the disease.

> I rather think that the hospital was less important in Irish or British life then than it is now. The hospital was associated a bit with the poor house. A working class family might have regarded going into the workhouse hospital as the end, as a risk.

Oral historians tend to be filled with regret over the unasked questions, the lanes of memory that interviewees push towards, but are not noticed until it is too late. When I met R.B., and asked how he was, he responded, with some deliberation: 'They tell me I'm not *too* bad for a man of my age, my blood pressure is ...'. Other mutual acquaintances noted that he always wore an overcoat and scarf, even in high summer. I ought to have asked him whether this early serious illness had left him with a concern that he was more vulnerable than others to illness that lasted beyond the teenage years he mentioned, and how that concern had impacted on the way he lived the rest of his long life.

His view that families in Belfast might regard entering the workhouse hospital (now Belfast City Hospital) as dangerous was echoed in an interview with veteran Belfast journalist James Kelly, born in 1911, who said that people he knew who were suffering from the flu – including his grandmother – were extremely reluctant to go to the workhouse hospital for treatment. 'Poor people did not want it to be noted that they died in the Union.' He recalled hearing that all the hospitals in Belfast were packed out. His family lived on the Falls Road, which led to two cemeteries, and he remembered black Belgian horses pulling hearses for days going to the hospitals with more cabs following them. Kelly's grandmother did indeed die in the Union hospital from the disease, but he could otherwise remember little else about it, other than that the schools were closed. 'I don't remember any of the kids getting it, although a lot of poor kids in St Paul's (his school) were in bare feet.' An able interviewee and eloquent raconteur who wrote a weekly column until his hundredth birthday, Kelly was clearly a little deflated that he could remember so little about the epidemic, but perhaps his family did not speak about it in front of the children.

Elizabeth Molloy was ninety-seven when interviewed in January 2007, and had lived in the Dublin satellite town of Lucan all her life. She described feeling scared and isolated when all her siblings and her parents fell ill with the flu. The house was cold, there was no food. She heard the 'ching of spurs' coming to the door, and felt relieved that help was at hand. It was her uncle – she called him a 'horse soldier' – returning from the war. He put her to bed on the settle, and when she woke he had lit the fire, made a stew, and was busy doling out quinine and whiskey to her sick family. They all recovered, and indeed most of them lived into their nineties. Soon afterwards a neighbour's twelve-year-old daughter died. This young girl had been a 'ministering angel' to Elizabeth's family and other neighbours, bringing them food and supplies, until she too became ill. She painted a vivid word picture of the girl's mother carrying the girl's body along the banks of the Grand Canal beseeching God to give her back. She pondered whether the Tontine Society had paid out much by way of a Christmas bonus during the influenza years. People made contributions each week towards a burial fund; at Christmas, the annual surplus was paid out. 'I don't think there was much left over that year.'[8]

Mrs Molloy's story was clearly very well polished. She had been a shopkeeper for many years, and several people acquainted with her told me I should interview her, as they had heard it. R.B. McDowell too has given an almost identical account to those of others, and even written it in his own memoirs; he was interviewed for a television documentary on personal experience of Spanish influenza, and the material he used there was again almost identical to the interview for this work. Other interviewees spoke hesitatingly, reflecting in the silences, as though it were the first time they had unearthed these memories of Spanish influenza from their long-term memory.[9]

Miss (Catherine) Doyle, at 104 the oldest of the people interviewed, was clearly distressed by the memory of the flu, although she insisted that it had not been so bad in St Mullins, the Co. Carlow area where she lived at the time. Born in 1903, she was fifteen when the flu came. 'Oh, that black flu, that was a terrible thing, you'd never forget that', she repeated several times. 'You'll have no trouble finding people to talk to you about that black flu.' It had made such an impression on her when she heard there was no Irish written history of the epidemic, she replied in staccato: 'I.am.speech.less.' She recalled her older brother falling ill, and his 'lovely head of curls left on the pillow'. Hair loss was such a common feature that newspaper advertisements offered products to remedy baldness caused by influenza. She professed to being fascinated with Spanish influenza because of her brother's experience with it.[10]

> Oh, the people went black. I didn't see any of them but some of them did. Oh, but it was a desperate flu. I was living in the Glebe at the time, in Carlow, near St Mullins. In any country places it was not as bad, it was the towns. In Graiguenamanagh a young pair got it and died, and the poor curate, he was found at some crossroad one night, he had gone out, he was delirious. He got it and went out. He was not dead. You see, it was never too bad outside Dublin, Dublin was bad, the towns were bad but the country was fairly good. 'A penny for the flu.' That was the word about it. Two died from it in the parish. Just two. One was a train driver; you see he went to fight it on his feet. There was no such thing as fighting that flu on your feet. In the country areas it was very very slight but in Dublin and the small towns, oh dear god, it was a different thing, oh dear. But then was not the Black Death worse?

She too considered influenza to be a sequela of the world war:

> I mean who knows, bodies not buried, I mean after wars, awful things happen in wars. Well they were blaming the war for the flu, you know the way people are just rotting abroad. I don't know, but it came anyhow ... Hickey I think was the doctor. He was too busy to be complaining. He had the work to do and that was it. The poor people used to go to the dispensary. That is one thing, people did not buy papers. You see, you could carry the disease with the papers.

Miss Doyle's family were farmers, so they had plenty of butter and eggs, and she said that they had no shortage 'except two ounces of tea or something'. Her brother Paddy remained sickly for a long time afterwards. He was fed whatever he was able to take. 'Gruel was supposed to be the best thing to feed him', she said, and it had to be 'cooked for ages and ages'. Several other interviewees mentioned gruel as a treatment for the invalids. She did not recall his being treated with whiskey or anything else; his throat was not sore, he felt nauseous and did not want any food.

> People went to Mass just the same, that did not keep people from going to Mass, that was their only hope. There was no hospital in Graiguenamanagh, there was one in New Ross. New Ross had it bad with flu, but they did not die. A young doctor in Dublin I said to him I thought what had really happened was that people tried to fight it on their feet. He said not at all, I was a young doctor at the time. I saw young strong men that came in the morning, they did not feel well in the morning, and that evening they were dead.

These three interviewees and many others associated the flu in some way with the First World War. Some thought that the flu had developed in the war, perhaps among rotting bodies in the trenches. Others believed that the returning soldiers brought it with them, and some suggested that the reason people were so vulnerable to the flu was because their bodies were weakened by war-associated deprivation.

Kathleen McMenamin, née O'Connor, caught influenza as a fourteen-year-old, while living in Rathmullan in Co. Donegal; she was 106 years old when she shared her influenza story with me. She, her mother and three brothers and two sisters all caught it. Her father did not. Her mother brought it into their house, having gone to help with nursing a neighbouring family, who were all ill. Kathleen said that at the time they understood it to have had its origins in the war, and some believed soldiers returning from war to be carriers and to have been partly responsible for the spread of influenza. Others thought it was an airborne virus with no connection with war. She thought that Rathmullan's use as a naval base during the war may have been a factor the unusually high incidence of influenza in Donegal in both 1918 and 1919. 'The fleet in Lough Swilly was under the control of Admiral Jellicoe so there were many sailors coming and going ashore at this time.' Her interview therefore offered an explanation for the puzzle on the high rate of death in Donegal. Many people in the village caught it and she recalled several deaths – a father and son in one family died on the same day, and two daughters in the same family died in England a year later. It affected young and old alike.

> My mother cared for us all while we were ill. I can remember that everyone with it complained of a terrible thirst and drank from jugs full of water. My youngest brother slept continuously for two full days without waking. Anyone prone to bronchitis or with a weak chest was likely to develop pneumonia from it and that usually proved fatal. My mother treated another of my brothers who had a weak chest by wrapping hot towels around his chest. I do not recall any visits to our home by a doctor or a nurse. There was no Mass in our church for a while and the school was closed also for a period. Weekly confessions were also cancelled for a period. People did not want to talk about it because it was so awful, and they dreaded the thought that it might come back again.[11]

Olive Vaughan, née Burgess, was born in 1910 in a nursing home in Baggot Street, and lived in Donnybrook as a child. She was eight at the time of the flu, and ninety-seven at the time of the interview, and was one of a family of eight children. She remembered people talking about people having the flu, and hoping that they would be alright, and the next thing was that person would be dead.

> It seemed to sweep through the world, really. Everyone was frightened of it. It happened after the war. Everybody seemed to associate it with the war and maybe the movement of population. It was not forgotten in those days; I remember the horror.

Mrs Vaughan said the emphasis of healthcare in those days was doctor-based. If people got sick, they called or visited a doctor, rather than going to a hospital or a clinic. She went to school at Sandford on Dublin's south side, but could not recall the school being closed because of the epidemic. She was not aware of being prevented from mixing with other children because of it. She expressed some surprise at not knowing more details about the flu, and considered that it may be because the adults in her family network used a type of code when they wanted to discuss things that were not considered appropriate for children to hear. This seems plausible as she could recall in detail other contemporaneous and earlier events, such as

British troops disembarking in Kingstown and marching through Donnybrook to the city centre in 1916, and also the end of the war in 1918. 'I remember the day the war was over carrying a flag with Queen Mary's photo on it.'[12]

Enid, (who asked to be referred to only by her first name) spoke of observing, as a seven-year-old, adults 'gathering in huddles to discuss this terrible illness that was going to kill more than were killed in the First World War'. But when it did come, it did not affect her or anybody she knew. Like other interviewees she suspected the reason she knew so little about the flu, despite having clear memories of other events at the time, was because her parents tried to prevent her hearing the more tragic stories. 'If there was tragedy the child might have been told to see if the kettle was boiling or something.' She pointed out the difference in news topics of conversation then compared to today, saying that as there was no media as such, the emphasis would focus on some subject and then move on very quickly. 'So there was this fear of flu, followed by interest in the armistice.' She thought the flu might have been forgotten because other events superseded it in importance; first the peace process, then the civil war and the breaking off of Ulster. 'The whole business of those years I think just swamped it.'[13]

Some interviewees thought that either their access or lack of access to good-quality food had a bearing on the extent to which their community suffered from the flu. Tommy Christian considered good food to be a factor in his family's recuperation. 'We had our own vegetables and grand spring water, that was in our favour.' Tommy was born in 1912, and has lived all his life on the Boston Road in Ardclough, north Kildare, which was then a rural area with a local economy dependent on agriculture about fifteen miles from the centre of Dublin. His father was a self-employed cobbler. As he spoke, he would leave long pauses, as he searched silently through the filing system of his memory for the right answers. Sometimes these answers were produced after an interval of some minutes or sometimes several weeks over a series of follow-up interviews. His mother, father, and he and his sister all got the flu.

> I was six years of age. We all got it, all the households, there was no one moving, even the doctor who was attending us got it. He was in Kill dispensary. The doctor had an old jalopy. He worked 24 hours round

the clock on his own, he could come at three o'clock in the morning. Then he got it himself, and we were plastered altogether. We were stricken down for three weeks maybe, and recovering afterwards was the most trying time of it. [A long pause.] The health services weren't too good at the time. It was a terrible disaster.[14]

Tommy said that there was a district nurse, but she was very old, and only had a bicycle to travel on. All the businesses and shops in his area were closed, masses suspended for a fortnight, and the landed estates were forced to hire women from the towns to do farm work. His memory of the difficulties local estates encountered in getting labourers to save crops during the epidemic is verified by an entry in the diary of Lord Cloncurry of Lyons estate, across the road from Tommy's house. The issue of a shortage of agricultural labour during the outbreak of influenza has also been mentioned in newspaper reports. The exceptionally wet weather in early autumn meant that crops were being saved later than usual.[15]

> The descendants of those people living now, they don't know how lucky they are that their parents weren't swept away with it ... [In response to a question about treatments for the flu] We were to make punch. We were to make sure that whatever you drank it was hot, the steam would help you, sure we could not swallow anything, our throats were so sore. And gruel, did you ever hear of gruel, it had an awful lot of responsibilities, this gruel. The O'Connors [a neighbouring farm family] brought us soup and stew, when they got back on their feet themselves. They would not have brought us down whiskey, that was a sin at that time. [In response to an inquiry about why it tends not to be remembered] There wasn't a terrible lot of talk about it afterwards. They were afraid to talk about it in case they could get it again. But a terrible lot of bad chests resulted from it. They were able to get them out of it, but a terrible lot of bad chests came from it. I don't think we were the same again for a long time ... it is a thing that will live with you for ever, that flu. People don't know much about it, there was never that much about it. Any survivors that got it would ever remember it. It was savage.[16]

Tommy offered without prompting that the flu was seldom spoken about once it was over. He reasoned that people were afraid to talk about it in case it came back again, as it had done twice before.

He had one apparently incongruous reference, when asked about where he thought the flu came from:

They blamed the war, the most of them, they put the blame on the war. There was the Asian flu, that was later. It was a mild thing compared to what we went through. Ships left Antwerp docks and they were infested with hoards of rats leaving for England. They blamed the rats [for the 'black flu'].

The rats reference may have been some speculation in newspapers – Tommy was an avid reader – that associated influenza with shipping; again this reference suggests a connection with plague. He recalled that there were a couple of deaths from influenza in Kill, a neighbouring parish with strong associations with Ardclough, and that a lot of people died in Naas. He said that it hit some places very hard, and that in places with big populations, one out of every ten people died.

While he survived, his mother died within a year of the epidemic. His father remarried, and moved to another house in the locality. Tommy and his sister were not part of the new household, remaining in their original home with an aunt caring for them. Even in later years, he had little contact with the step-family. An RTE television team, which was filming a documentary about his memory of Spanish influenza, was, by an odd twist of fate, with him the day his younger half-brother died. He insisted on continuing the filming, saying: 'Sure what would that have to do with me?' There was a slight touch of anger in his voice, but perhaps that was a cover for a complicated sadness. Perhaps the informed watchers imagined the tear in his eye. Sometimes the oral historian should present what they see and leave it to the reader to interpret, bearing in mind – as Mark Cave has written – that emotion is a big part of truth, particularly if it has been formed in times of crisis.[17] It was not until a second interview that Tommy associated his mother's death as being caused by post-influenzal malaise; she had never fully recovered her health after contracting the disease. This revelation was a surprise to the next generation of his family. Mrs Christian's death was not registered, so it is not possible to confirm her cause of death. Tommy's memory about other details relating to influenza in his locality had shown not only remarkable detail but exceptional accuracy when cross-checked, so there seems little reason to doubt this association.

As this strain of influenza seemed to target young adults, Tommy's story of losing a parent and having family circumstances drastically

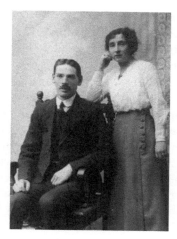

Figure 15 James and Margaret Delaney, 1915.

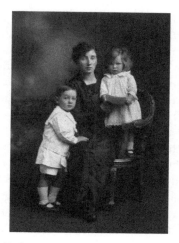

Figure 16 Margaret Delaney with their two children Denis and Rebecca.

changed by influenza is a common one. Nellie Tubridy, née Marrinan, was born in the spring of 1919; her mother had caught influenza and gone into premature labour in Sligo, where Nellie's father was stationed with the Royal Irish Constabulary. Her mother died. Weighing just over two pounds and given little chance of survival, the tiny infant was brought by train, cart and on foot, resting at strategic intervals in houses where the family had arranged for fires to be stoked up along the way for her arrival, to her father's sister Ellen Corry's home in Kilmacduane, Co. Clare, where she was raised as part of her aunt's family. As a result of their smaller body mass, underweight premature babies lose heat quickly. Nellie's oldest son Jim Tubridy said that for many weeks, until she was better able to maintain her own body temperature, his aunt and her husband took turns to sleep with her on the settle bed beside a constantly burning fire. Given the care required to keep such a tiny infant alive even with modern medical equipment, her survival showed great nursing skills. She was a bright and engaging woman who lived into her eighties and often spoke of her first adventure in life: 'You know I was only the size of a bag of sugar?'[18]

When James Delaney, a Laois-born constable working with the Dublin Metropolitan Police (DMP) at Lad Lane in Dublin, died from pneumonia after apparently recovering from influenza and returning to work, it had long reaching consequences for his family, his grand-daughter Ann Delaney Burke told me. Their lives had quite a different path from what they might have expected, had James lived. He had no pension. To support her family, his wife Maggie opened a cake shop on Kimmage Cross Road, Dublin, next to her brother's butcher's shop: 'I presume she needed to earn an income of her own, even though her father and brothers owned quite a few properties all over Dublin as well as running a business.'

Ann said her father Denis seemed to know very little about his father, other than these facts, and that Becky, her aunt, just one year old when James died, was killed by scarlatina on 18 May 1923 in Cork Street fever hospital. Denis and his mother Maggie lived with her two brothers and father, and moved house several times, eventually settling in Simmonstown, Co. Kildare, where she was born and lives today. Given the losses of his father and sister – and that Maggie's mother Rebecca O'Keeffe McBennett had died in the Russian pandemic of the 1890s – it is not surprising to learn that he was cosseted as a child. The only sport he was allowed to play was cricket. 'He was very precious to them.' As an adult, Ann says that Denis maintained a silence about James, and his side of the family. 'These were the facts that I grew up with, no stories, no memories, not even an image apart from a wedding photograph that lay hidden in a drawer for many years.'[19]

As an only child, she had a close sense of family, but few relations, and longed to hear more about her grandfather and his people. She came to realise that his death had had a profound effect on Denis, who could be 'difficult', and that it was something he could not fully share. So the influenza loss fascinated her all the more. One way in which it seemed to be expressed was his hatred of uniforms. She often thought he blamed the uniform for his father's death, which, given that James returned to work with the DMP after apparently recovering, was not illogical:

> My father's connection with his paternal family was very strange and private, he never spoke much of them, although he did tell me that as a child he was sent down to Derryguile (the County Laois family home of James) to stay with his grandparents during the summer with ten shillings pinned to his vest. One other occasion I remember, he drove myself and my mother down to Mountmellick (when I was maybe ten) and went as far as a small laneway and stopped the car. He pointed and said that his father was born there. We went no further and the car was turned around and we came home.

It will come as no surprise to the reader to hear Ann has developed an interest in tracing her grandfather's family:

> He was the eldest boy, two of his sisters went to Philadelphia and made lives for themselves there, two sisters and two younger brothers stayed in Derryguile or nearby, married and raised families. I wonder did my Dad know that he had twenty-six first cousins and if he did why did we never meet? The relations I found in my research have been open and kind beyond belief, they have sent me photos I would never have otherwise, they have written wonderful letters and told me about my lost family, I have been shown graves and cottages, but there are huge gaps, never to be filled. Another family member on my grandmother's side told me how sociable Maggie was and how she loved to entertain, yet she was left a widow at thirty, she wore black or dark colours all her life (I know as her clothes remained in her wardrobe after her death and I used to dress up in them as a child). She never remarried or lived independently. Sadly, I never knew her as she died just three weeks before I was born. I live in the same house she

died in and for that I am thankful, but if her husband had survived, that might not have been. They surely would have lived elsewhere and maybe had more children. My Dad would not have been the sole focus of his grandfather, two uncles and a mother's life. Perhaps my life would also have been different. I might not be living here, who can say?

Dr James Walsh was a former Dean of the Faculty of Public Health Medicine in the Royal College of Physicians, and former deputy chief medical officer, Department of Health. Dr Walsh was born in 1923. He recalled talk of the epidemic when he was growing up, and analysed it with hindsight, using the expertise of his work as a public health specialist.[20] He spoke of the dread of Spanish influenza in his community and among the medical profession even as he was growing up in the 1920s and 1930s. He grew up in New Ross in a medical family; his grandfather had been the senior doctor in the Houghton Hospital in New Ross. He professed a fascination with the epidemic, partly because it had a familial connection through his grandfather's work, and partly because he became a public health specialist. Now, several years later, I wonder whether his early knowledge of the 1918–19 influenza pandemic shaped his medical career, leading him to public health.

> It always fascinated me that even the world war, which had been awful, four years of murder and slaughter, and in which lots of local men had been killed, because we were still part of the United Kingdom then, that that seemed to have less of an impact than the Spanish flu. They were particularly in a state of fear because so many young people died. The other thing that affected them was the suddenness of the symptoms. An individual could be well on Monday, sick on Tuesday and dead on Wednesday. This really terrified them. And then mumbo jumbo started off, as always, everything becomes mysterious. Because they mostly died of bronchial pneumonia they became cyanosed, and not alone did the flu kill them, but they turned blue or black before they died. This was serious stuff. There was also a feeling of the impotence of the medical profession. The public was aware that apart from treating symptoms, they didn't really do anything.

Walsh's grandfather, Dr Michael Walsh, believed that whiskey had anti-viral properties; he claimed to have poured whiskey into the Houghton's influenza patients, and as a result of that, the Houghton was reputed to have had far higher survival rates than the local district hospital. James Walsh suggested that a more plausible reason was that the kind of people who went to the Houghton were middle-class, reasonably prosperous farmers, whose nutrition would have been good, whereas the fever hospital's patients tended to be poorer people. He considered it obvious that the world war was what spread the disease:[21]

> For four years men had been in trenches, sometimes up their knees in water, and surrounded by rats and lice. Then they were asked to climb out of the hole and charge. Given that the ground was turn up by huge artillery, the entire land around was torn to shreds, who knows what. Disturbing land and old viruses is not a good idea … Apart from the horrible conditions when it ended they were dispatched to all parts of the world. The spread of the disease would have been considerably curtailed if they had not been dispatched to all corners of the world, America, Australia, New Zealand, Britain.

Dr Walsh believed that the medical profession suffered from a sense of failure and panic in the period immediately after the pandemic, because their understanding of medical science had been insufficient to deal with the disease, and that this forced responses which eventually turned into the WHO influenza-monitoring systems that exist today.

> What happened then was a shadow was cast over not just the ordinary public but the medical profession as well, that if we got another virus like this, what were we going to do? The WHO [World Health Organization] [later] set up sentinel virus laboratories which look at the strains each year, and what effect that has is when a new strain of the virus appears it is a race between getting a vaccine and the wider spread of the disease. The [Spanish] flu virus had the effect of damaging the epithelium of the lungs. There was very little could be done for them. There was no penicillin of course. One of the arguments for today is that now we have antibiotics which are very effective against these pyogenic organisms – pus forming, they cough up pussy sputum … The answer to flu epidemics is vaccination with a relevant vaccine given on time. The interesting thing is that they have noted for the present flu [he refers to the 2009 Influenza A H1N1 pandemic] that people born before 1925, some people say later, do not get the disease, do not get the disease or get it in a mild form. We [healthcare workers] should all be honest and say we know very little about the flu virus.

I would subscribe to [a theory] that when a virus appears, it just doesn't disappear, it usually harbours in an animal or bird host, and then it reappears when a susceptible host appears before it. In other words, it is almost like a military strategy. And that brings us to an interesting point, if people of a certain age don't get the virus, what virus was around before 1925, but there is reasonable evidence to suggest that the virus was caused by the H1N1, that's why they have immunity, and that it came from the Spanish flu. I am talking about a virus that is so clever that it stays in an animal host until it spots a susceptible population, and then, bang, it hits again. If that is the case, that the virus which caused the Mexican flu is very similar if not the same as the one that caused the Spanish flu, then we have to be very careful, and ... it may become very virulent, and begin killing people.

Many other interviewees spoke of whiskey being used as a treatment and as a prophylactic measure, including Tommy Christian and Elizabeth Molloy, who were both fed whiskey or whiskey punch as sick children. Raphael Sieve's father, Albert, believed he saved his own younger brother Harry's life when he caught the Spanish flu as a twenty-year-old. The family lived in Lombard Street West, off Dublin's Clanbrassil Street. Believing Harry's life to be particularly threatened as he was in that young-adult age group that Spanish flu seemed to target, Mr. Sieve senior kept his brother indoors and constantly mildly drunk for a couple of weeks until he recovered. 'He fed him whiskey and alcohol and saved him that way.' Raphael heard the talk about flu as a child, and when he caught a cold they would tell the story. John Fitzgerald's father, also John, worked in Ryan's pub in Dun Laoghaire. He caught the flu and was brought to St Michael's Hospital, where he remembered thirteen dying in one night from the flu. The publican took him in 'biscuit' brandy and the father reckoned that saved him.[22]

An interview on a separate project pointed me obliquely to a good reason for the failure of historians or public memory to the influenza as a significant public health event. While working on an oral history of labour project, I interviewed Stella McConnon Larkin, granddaughter of the Liverpool-born Irish trade union leader James Larkin. As Stella spoke of her grandfather and father's diligent commitment to improving the housing and wages of the labouring poor of Dublin, she revealed that her mother Anna Moore Larkin had been one of ten children born to a family in the infamous tenements in the centre of Dublin, and the only one who survived beyond the age of five. The discussion of the syndemic conditions which caused high rates of death among the children of the city's poor in the statistics chapter are revealed at family level in the awfulness of what happened to Stella's mother's family. Her testimony shows the real power of oral history to add human experience of suffering to the dry bones of statistics. She had been told that some of the family had died in the flu epidemic, and others had died from 'the diseases of childhood that killed so many others at the time'. This family, the Moores, lived in a one room of a house in the centre of Dublin, at 34 Marlborough Street. Civil registration and Glasnevin Cemetery records enabled me to find that four of the Moore children died from infectious disease between 1911 and 1918: infant diarrhoea, measles and in November 1918, four-year-old Mary Moore died from influenza at the height of the second wave. Two others had died by the time of the 1911 census. It was Stella's thoughtful discussion of the difficulties of living in these conditions that suggested to me that the syndemic conditions – a cacophony of diseases of which influenza was just another noise – may partly explain the failure of the 1918–19 influenza to leave a significant impact on public memory in Ireland, even though families clearly remembered their losses privately. In the 1910s, children under five would typically account for one fifth of the annual deaths; part of the reason for this high toll was the appalling living conditions of Dublin's poor, where one third of families lived in one room tenements, sharing an outside privy with the other families.[23] In these cramped and unhygienic rooms, child death was commonplace; many died from marasmus and tuberculosis, and childhood diseases like measles and scarlet fever would spread rapidly.

Another potential interviewee, who had been suggested by a colleague as a reliable witness, said that although she would have been delighted to be able to help, the flu would not have affected her family as they were well-to-do. When pressed further, she revealed that her father was a chauffeur for the Guinness brewing company; the family lived in Bride Street in Dublin city centre, a short walk from tenements, but in her view a different world. She associated the influenza pandemic with overcrowded housing and conditions of poverty in the nearby tenements, which led to many dying from disease. Some interviewees tended to conflate the brief influenza pandemic with the longer tuberculosis epidemic. Sometimes they would contact me to find out whether their relation had died from influenza, and when I returned with a death certificate citing tuberculosis they seemed to know that already. Even almost a hundred years later, they hoped to find that the relation had died from influenza rather than from tuberculosis, with its socially negative connotations.

Perhaps surprisingly, only one of the people interviewed for this project suggested that the disease was linked to privations the Irish suffered as a result of oppression by the British imperialist system. Sister Theresa, a Dominican nun, was born in 1912 on an island in Lough Reagh near Lanesboro, the eighth of ten children. She does not recall the flu happening at the time but was told about it later.

> My godmother, a neighbour, a young girl of 18, she died from the flu, I don't remember it. On the island, Inchéanaí, during the troubles, an old house was used as a hospital. I had a first cousin, they lived in Co. Roscommon, she died of the flu, eighteen years of age. The country was very poor at that time; England had crushed them so much. The people were very poor and undernourished. It was no wonder that they all died.[24]

Many considered that poverty, for whatever reason, made people more prone to the disease. Sister Wilfrid Callanan, born in 1916, thought that influenza affected poor people worse than the better off. She lived in Patrickswell, Co. Limerick, with her family in a small house.

> We were just after the big war, and there must have been an awful lot of shortages. Families were large. Six would be a small family. My mother spoke about the flu. I was only two years old in 1918 when the flu was raging. It took my uncle Paddy, my father's brother, and many others too. I have asked three or four people here [colleagues in the nursing home], and they have memories of losing people; they said 'my poor father was taken and there was no man to look after the farm, and us girls had to go and work' or something like that. My mother said that nearly every family lost somebody to the flu ... I think it was that the people were worn out from the war. You could not get a drop of tea. In the last war we lived on porridge. Around where I was there was a lot of working class people. That might be why [it hit us so hard]. The world was a different place then. Our aunt [whose husband died from the flu] had to go out and work, she worked on an ambulance. They used to send round an ambulance and it had to have a man and a woman on it. She had small children at the time, two girls and a boy.

The youngest girl died at 12 of tuberculosis. They fumigated their room with a sulphur candle. I connect the flu with that war [the First World War]. The soldiers who were coming back, they would have brought it. They brought back all sorts of things.[25]

Some associated catching the flu with travelling on trains or working for train companies. Miss Doyle spoke of an outbreak of influenza among railway workers based at Graiguenamanagh. John Ralph, a farmer from Tombrack in north Wexford, died from influenza on 13 October 1918, leaving a widow and five children; his family believe John may have caught flu when he went to Dublin on the train on business. His eldest son Joe was then a boy of eleven; Joe's wife, Cissie, recalled that Joe was so traumatised by his father's death that he never spoke about it. Some years ago she discovered that Joe's father was buried on the same day that her own mother's first husband was buried, having also died from the disease, in another north Wexford area, Monageer. Margaret Deacon's uncle, Sam Williamson, born in 1885, was a married builder living in Kilcormac Rectory, who died from influenza; Margaret's mother used to say that her brother Sam went from Enniscorthy to Dublin on the train on building business and came back in his coffin.[26]

Very few of the interviewees mentioned any connection between religion or spirituality and the flu, even though many of those interviewed were religious people; only one of the interviewees spoke of having given up religious belief, later in life. Mrs Molloy spoke of the neighbour appealing to God to give her daughter back. Eileen 'Bab' Davitt spoke of the superstitions about the flu, and of how unaware her north Wexford community was of the association between the several influenza deaths over the length of three miles of road. Her grandmother and great-aunt nursed another Knockreagh family, the Lancasters, when they were sick with the flu. They were concerned their act of charity would bring the influenza to their own families, so they consulted the parish priest based four miles away in Ferns. 'The priest promised them that they would not bring it to their own families, and they did not.' The two often spoke about how God had kept the priest's promise to them. Two of the Lancaster family, the mother Kate, then in her late fifties, and a teenage son died. A younger son, Denis, aged thirteen, was also ill. 'When the older boy died, Mr. [Denis] Lancaster prayed: "For God's sake,

leave me one son." Mrs. Lancaster died the next day.' Bab said that
while her mother and aunt knew that the Lancasters' flu was dangerous and risky for them as nurses, they did not know that other
close neighbours were also dying from the disease at that time, that
along two miles of sparsely populated country road at least six people
had died. 'We did not know about Mr Ralph, for example, or John
Walsh in Tombrack, or the Milnes in Clohamon dying from the
flu.'[27] The Milnes she referred to were a husband and wife living in
Castlequarter, Clohamon, about two miles further along the road
towards Bunclody; both died during the epidemic and their teenage
son and daughter were sent to be cared for by two different branches
of the family.

Help for influenza victims from neighbours and landlords was a
common theme. Elizabeth Molloy, Bab Davitt and Tommy Christian
recounted the help they received from neighbours. Nellie O'Toole,
who lived in Rathvilly, Co. Carlow, credited Lord Rathdonnell of
Lisnaveagh with keeping the people of the village alive during the
influenza epidemic. Born in 1908, she had five older brothers and one
younger sister; the family lived in Phelan's row, Rathvilly. Everyone
in the family apart from her caught the flu; she claims never to have
caught the flu or even a cold in her life.[28]

> My parents caught it, not so bad, they were all in bed at different
> stages. One of the brothers who got sick first, Jimmy, he beat his
> head against the wall, he was so sick. Lord Rathdonnell kept the
> people alive, he sent down a man with two milk churns full of thick
> soup. I used to help the man with the soup put it out. I left it on
> the step, outside each house, they could see me coming through
> the window. Of course, I brought it into our own house. No-one in
> Phelan's row died. Yet someone from every house was sick with the
> flu. We lived in number eleven, my father's sister lived in number
> twelve, my uncle the cobbler lived in number one. Aunt Abby got
> sick from the flu, yet she still lived to 105. The soup helped; other-
> wise a lot of people would have died. The milk churns [of soup] were
> lovely. You just turned on the tap and it came out. I did not hear
> about other places getting it, although maybe there was something
> about someone in Tullow getting it before us. They said the Asia flu
> has come to Ireland, and to watch out for it.

Nellie said that if they wanted the doctor, for the influenza patients,
the dispensary doctor in Rathvilly would come down. The doctor gave

them pills or medicine for the flu, and Jimmy was given an injection for the pain in his head. Unlike other doctors, he did not suggest treating the flu with poultices. 'He [the doctor] did not give anything strong.' Jimmy took several months to recover, and lost a lot of weight. He was a teenager at the time.

> Everything was closed down, it was a deserted village, no-one was able to work. The soup came down around 11 or 12 o'clock to the village, brought down in a phaeton from the big house. It was not cold weather, there was no waiting around in the rain for the soup. It would be to Dublin they would have been moved if anyone was very bad, and I did not hear of anybody being moved to hospital. You just had to stay in bed. I was running around, I was the only one who did not get it in the village, it was deserted.

Nellie's mother was a community reader; she would assemble a group of neighbours and family and read news from an evening newspaper Nellie believed it was the *Evening Herald*, 'definitely not the *Evening Mail*'; it seems likely that the community in this way had good warning of the pandemic's imminent arrival and the medical advice to keep well nourished, with plenty of fluids, and to stay in bed until it had passed.

Some families hardly knew the pandemic was happening even when they lived in areas where people were ill and dying around them. Dean Thomas Salmon, a former dean of Christ Church Cathedral, Dublin said that as children, his family were kept in relative isolation in their Dublin home. Born in 1913, in the middle of a family of eight, he stressed that his family were anxious to keep knowledge of both the world war and the Irish revolutionary period away from the children. 'We were kept out of it as much as possible. We were all educated at home ... so we would not have mixed with the flu.' Rosalind Andrews, née Knoles, whose family lived on Haddon Road, Dublin, at the time, could not recall much about the flu, although she had a very clear memory of a family friend dying when the *Leinster* was torpedoed. 'My father had to identify him; that is clear, but the flu is not.' She had a vague impression that some of her family – she was one of seven siblings – were in bed with flu, and mentions but does not associate as being the same disease that her brother caught – 'bad pneumonia' – twice when he was in the field artillery in France. 'In my young days there were wars and shootings every night and rebellions there were so many other things happening that it was probably forgotten about.' Florrie Taylor, née Bagnall, was born in 1913, and was living on the family farm in Westmeath when the influenza epidemic occurred. She was five at the time of the flu, and had many other memories from around that time, including British soldiers calling to take hay; she was attending school, and did not recall it being closed during the pandemic, and has no memories of people being ill with influenza.[29]

Olive Rynhart, who lived in the north Wexford village of Ferns, reported that the chapel and church bells never seemed to stop ringing at that time.[30] Many other interviewees mentioned the constant ringing of church bells for funerals at the time, indicating the deep effect the pandemic had on their communities.

Reports of multiple deaths within one family from influenza were a common feature of the interviews. Anne Shankey shared her mother's memories of her mother's sister, brother and father all dying from Spanish flu. They were laid out in the front room of the family home in Leeson Park Avenue for some time as there was a delay at the undertakers. The family believed it was because there was an industrial dispute at Nichols undertakers. Nichols' records indicate that the strike was over by the time Richard Bailey, a plumber and businessman, and his son Robert and daughter Gertie died; the delay may have been at the cemetery, as during the peak weeks some cemeteries had to queue burials. Nichols also appear to have staggered the payments for the three burials, perhaps to ease the financial burden on Mrs Bailey; burying that many dead was an expensive business.[31] The Baileys were another of the many families who had their economic circumstances changed by the loss of the family income earner. At one stage, Mrs Bailey was asked if she wanted to send the remaining children to one of the Protestant orphanages, but she would not agree, as she was afraid she would not get them back, and like Ann Delaney Burke's grandmother, took control of providing the family income. Mary McNally Sheil whose mother and grandmother had nursed 'black flu' patients in Liverpool – her grandmother died from the disease – was told by a civil servant colleague that his father, mother and four siblings had died from the flu when he was fourteen, leaving only himself and his six-year-old sister. They were buried so quickly he did not even know where they were buried.[32]

Séamus Claffey ran a hardware and undertakers' business in Ferbane, Co. Offaly. His father was an undertaker during the epidemic and told Séamus that business had been very good during that time; the business archives only run from 1928:[33]

> There was a simple rule. If you got the flu you went to bed and if you did not, you died. My father was an undertaker. He buried them, I suppose we shouldn't say in their dozens. Say whole families died, because they did not obey the rules. It is the same today, if you get the flu. The strong people who were the ones who died, the men did not obey the rules. A local school teacher, Mr. Henry, was the first person to die in Ferbane from the Big Flu.

Séamus cited the story of a named man from Pullagh who was one of a group of thirty-six Irish soldiers who were demobilised after the war and were coming back through England. Nineteen of the thirty-six died on their way through England on the way home, and it was understood that they had died from flu. 'My mother used to say demobbed soldiers brought back the flu with them.' During the pandemic a man came in and asked his father the time for a funeral. His father told him he couldn't give him a time, there were so many on. At the height of the Claffey funeral business there were fifty funerals a year, an average of one a week, but 'during the Big Flu there were several a day. Sin an scéal, heads of house died, fathers died, they got the story pretty fast, you go to bed or you die, when poor Mr Henry died. I suppose people learned from that. My father told me an awful lot of people died in Clonfanla, near Clonmacnoise'.

Undertakers and timber merchants were some of the businesses that did well out of others' misfortune. Dr Hugh Byrne said that his father, who was the son of a timber merchant, told him that the coffins were stacked eighteen high with bodies in them in the mortuary in what was to become St James' Hospital, then St Kevin's (the Dublin Union hospital). He had heard that the business thrived by supplying timber for coffins during the Spanish flu. One of the undertakers they supplied was Fanagan's.[34]

Some interviews support newspaper reports and statistics which point to certain occupations, particularly those dealing with the public, left people more vulnerable to catching the flu. Lena Higgins, born in Sallins, Co. Kildare in 1916, became extremely distressed as she recalled the deaths of her father's two brothers (who worked in shops in Arklow, Co. Wicklow) and of her father's two nephews and a niece, children of shopkeepers on Main Street in Gorey, Co. Wexford. An account of the deaths of these children, from a family named Doran, is in the Wexford newspapers. Mrs Doran, sister of the interviewee's father, caught a severe attack of influenza but survived. The Gogartys, a family with hardware and general merchant shops in Co. Kildare towns of Celbridge and Naas, also lost five family members to the disease over the space of three months, in Canada and Belgium as well as Ireland. The death of James Delaney, a DMP constable, demonstrated not only the risk presented to the police force by their close contact with the public, but also the way that influenza deaths could alter the structure of families.[35]

Others spoke of social distancing during the pandemic. Mary Anne Rowsome, born in 1909, lived then in Tomsallagh, Ferns, Co. Wexford. 'People would not go into the houses, or they would not come into contact with anyone who had it. A lot of people died from it. The schools were closed, but Mass was not cancelled.' She recalled there being bonfires to celebrate the end of the First World War, but said that people were afraid of catching the flu at the celebrations. This social distancing may have been effective, as nobody in her family caught flu; she was one of ten children.[36]

Fear about the pandemic lingered for many years after, as Dr Walsh reported. Several interviewees spoke of their parents wrapping them up in very warm clothes 'in case they caught the flu'; during the 1920s, buses were disinfected during influenza outbreaks, which some interviewees indicated was a hangover of the fear from the 1918–19 influenza pandemic.

These interviews represent an enduring line, a direct connection to the experience of the Spanish influenza pandemic in Ireland. They help to document the legacy of the impact, and to indicate the trauma suffered by the Irish during the pandemic. They also seem to show that the oral history interview, used to create a new source for the study of this pandemic, can be a two-way process. Not only does it provide the historian with a rich source of material that is not otherwise possible to access, but it also provides the subject – the interviewee, who in these circumstances could be viewed as a victim, with a schema to make sense of a traumatic event in their childhood that seemed inexplicable, irrational, nebulous and localised, until set into the context of the national and international narrative of the pandemic.

As a collective body, these interviews enable us to understand the evidence about the pandemic in the earlier chapters in a different way, through human memory and interpretation. They show that Spanish influenza, far from being a forgotten pandemic, still has a presence in popular memory, and was viewed by those who had first-hand experience of it, or whose family had suffered traumas, as being 'unforgettable', even if the epidemic was forgotten or not considered worthy of attention by Irish historians. They indicate that there was an expectancy that the flu was coming, and that there was an individual and collective fear of the flu, both before it arrived and during it, possibly fuelled by advance warnings of its arrival in the newspapers, and that there was little confidence in the LGB's competence to deal with it. They show that primary healthcare came from the LGB's agents, the medical officers of health, who Tommy Christian and others have verified literally worked around the clock to care for the ill, at great personal risk, and that the public held them in high esteem as a result of their diligence. They reveal the human tragedies, the orphaned children and widowed spouses, the parents who lost one or more of their children in almost inexplicable circumstances, the changing economic circumstances of families as a result of the death or loss of health of a breadwinner. They also document the survival stories – the children whose health was so threatened by influenza that they were not expected to live through the night, but who lived at least into their nineties, out-surviving other members of the family, including those who did not catch the disease. They indicate that Sinn Féin's attempt to frame the effects of the disease on Irish nationalists as another example of British injustice, mentioned in another chapter, did not seem to make a lasting impression on the collective memory. They also show that responses to caring for patients seemed to come, not from the government, but from community initiatives, reflected in the efforts of neighbours to nurse the ill at great personal risk, or in the foresight of landlords like Lord Rathdonnell who provided nourishing food for those not able to provide for themselves. This last point is possibly the strongest one, which these interviews as a collective body of evidence prove: in the absence of any grand strategic plan to deal with the flu emerging from the offices of the

LGB, or of the development of an effective medicine or vaccine by the medical profession and their ancillaries, the best weapons people had to fight the flu were the help of neighbours and good home nursing.

Notes

1 Richard Collier, *The Plague of the Spanish Lady* (London: Atheneum, 1974).
2 Mark Honigsbaum, *Living with Enza* (Basingstoke: Palgrave Macmillan, 2009).
3 Niall Johnson, *Britain and the 1918–19 Influenza Pandemic: a Dark Epilogue* (Abingdon: Routledge), pp. 162–3.
4 Joanna Bornat, 'Oral history as a social movement: reminiscence and older people', in Robert Perks, and Alistair Thomson, eds, *The Oral History Reader* (London: Routledge, 1998), pp. 189–205. Charles Rosenberg, *Explaining Epidemics and Other Studies in the History of Medicine* (Cambridge: Cambridge University Press, 1992), p. 283.
5 For a further discussion of the ability of the elderly to provide accurate and useful recall, see Paul Thompson, *The Voice of the Past – Oral History* (Oxford: Oxford University Press, 2000).
6 Trevor Lummis, 'Structure and validity in oral evidence', in Robert Perks and Alistair Thomson, eds, *The Oral History Reader* (Abingdon: Routledge, 2014, third edn), pp. 273–83.
7 Interview with RB McDowell, Trinity, College Dublin, in December 2006. No mention of the disease was found in the Trinity College muniments.
8 Interview with Elizabeth Molloy, Lucan, Co. Dublin, 16 January 2007.
9 R.B. McDowell, *Crisis and Decline: the Fate of the Southern Unionists* (Dublin: Lilliput Press, 1997). McDowell was interviewed for *Outbreak*, a documentary series on disease produced by Janet Gallagher, RTE 1, 2 June 2009.
10 Interview with Catherine Doyle, Lucan, Co. Dublin, 23 February 2007.
11 Personal communication with Kathleen McMenamin, née O'Connor, Rathmullen, Co. Donegal, October 2010.
12 Interview with Olive Vaughan, née Burgess, in Brabazon nursing home, St John's Road, Sandymount, Dublin, 22 January 2007.
13 Interview with Enid, who did not wish to be further identified; name and address with author; interviewed in Dublin, July 2007.
14 Interviews with Tommy Christian, Ardclough, Co. Kildare, 12 April, 2007, and subsequent communications. *Outbreak*, produced by Janet Gallagher, RTE 1, 2 June 2009.

15 Lord Cloncurry's diary for 1918 and 1919. In private hands. Entry for Monday 28 October 1918. 'At Lyons, dry day all hands at lifting and pitting potatoes in Skeagh. Nine of the workmen away from work, mainly influenza. Ten women and girls from Celbridge picking potatoes.' For discussion of autumn weather causing delays in saving crops, see *Kilkenny People*, 19 October 1918.

16 Some medical doctors placed emphasis on purging the bowels as part of the influenza treatment régime. See Chapter 5.

17 Mark Cave, 'What remains – reflections on crisis oral history', in Perks and Thompson, eds, *The Oral History Reader*, pp. 92–103.

18 Interview with Jim Tubridy, Cooraclare, Co. Clare, 28 November 2008.

19 Email communication with Ann Delaney Burke, 6 February 2017.

20 Interview with Dr James Walsh, former dean of the faculty of public health at the Royal College of Physicians, and former deputy chief medical officer, Department of Health, on 9 December 2009.

21 Whiskey was frequently used as the treatment of choice by doctors, who sometimes also used it prophylactically. See also Chapters 4 and 5.

22 Telephone communication with John Fitzgerald, Co. Meath, 31 March 2008.

23 Charles Cameron, *Report Upon the State of Public Health and the Sanitary Work Performed in Dublin During the Year 1919*. (Dublin: Dublin Corporation, 1920), p. 94.

24 Interview with Sr Theresa, Sancta Maria Dominican nursing home, Cabra Road, 8 March 2007.

25 Interview with Sr Wilfrid Callanan, Sancta Maria Dominican nursing home, Cabra Road, Dublin, 8 March 2007.

26 Interview with Margaret Deacon, Enniscorthy, Co. Wexford, 13 July 2007.

27 Interview with Eileen Bab Davitt, 8 July 2008.

28 Interview with Nellie O'Toole, Merrion Row, Dublin, 30 September 2008. Surviving the flu turned Nellie into something of a media celebrity in her later years; her story appeared also in Turtle Bunbury's *Vanishing Ireland* (Dublin: Hachette Books Ireland, 2006); she was also interviewed on RTE's *Pat Kenny Show* and on the RTE television documentary series on survivors of Spanish influenza and other diseases, *Outbreak*.

29 Interview with Rosalind Andrews, née Knoles, Blackheath Park, Dublin, 9 July 2007. Interview with Florrie Taylor and with Dean Salmon at Brabazon Nursing Home, Sandymount, Dublin, 23 January 2007.

30 Interview with Cissie Ralph, Ferns, Co. Wexford, 20 August 2009. Telephone communication with Olive Rynhart, Killoggy Castle, Ferns, Co. Wexford, 20 February 2007.

31 Telephone communication with Anne Shankey, Dublin, 31 March 2008. National Archives business records series 19/2/8, J. and E. Nichols

daybook for 1916–1919, lists burials for the Bailey family of Leeson Park Avenue on 9 January, 15 March and 5 June 1919, but newspaper death notices and the death certificate entry confirm the family story that all three died within a short time period.

32 Interview with Mary McNally Sheil, Rathcoole, Co. Dublin, 20 April 2007.

33 Interview with Seamus Claffey, Ferbane, Co. Offaly, 17 November 2007. The business records of the family undertaking and hardware business only run from 1928.

34 Telephone communication with Hugh Byrne, 30 March 2008. Fanagan's business records for this time do not survive.

35 Interview with Lena Higgins in Larchfield Nursing Home, Naas, Co. Kildare, 5 July 2007. Interview with Catherine Boylan, Celbridge, Co. Kildare, 20 November 2008. The Gogarty tombstones are in St Corban's cemetery, Naas, and Donaghcumper cemetery, Celbridge. Interview with Ann Burke, Simmonstown, Celbridge, 6 February 2007.

36 Interview with Mary Anne Rowsome in the Moyne Nursing Home, Enniscorthy, Co. Wexford, 13 July 2007.

8

Influenza as a political tool

To describe the 1910s as an evolutionary decade for Irish society is something of an understatement. The involvement of significant numbers of Irish people in the world war and a rush of mood-altering domestic events – the 1913 Dublin strike and lockout, the deferral of Home Rule, the 1916 rebellion and the death on hunger strike of nationalist prisoner Thomas Ashe – made transformative calls on loyalty. In the wake of the 'failed' 1916 rebellion, the nationalist movement reorganised, understanding that public outrage at the execution of rebellion leaders pointed to other ways than military tactics of achieving their aims, and developing more confidence as it became clear that their popular support was increasing. The Irish Volunteers displayed this growing confidence through public marching and drilling; alarmed at such brashness, the authorities arrested and court martialled many under the regulations for Defence of the Realm Acts passed to protect British domestic interests in wartime, as William Murphy explains so thoroughly in his history of political internment in the period. Murphy argues that protest in prisons became the most radical and effective form of nationalism by 1917 and 1918.[1] Advanced nationalists made full use of the opportunities provided by prison conflict to ram home their political message through propaganda. Carefully penned stories of injustice and deprivation could be mightier than the bullet.

Ben Novick and Virginia Glandon discuss the methods that advanced nationalist propagandists used to drive the engine of the Irish revolution: for them, propagandists effectively harnessed newspaper columns, ballad sheets, election material, or speeches and performances, to ensure that their version of events reached the public consciousness. The National Council of Sinn Féin continually encouraged members around Ireland to publicise their activities through both the advanced nationalist newspapers and the letter columns of the daily papers. One pamphlet produced for Sinn Féin cumainn (Irish for 'branches') in 1918 declared: 'There is not a week passes, but some incident occurs in every county which could be turned to account for driving home the lesson that the country must look to Sinn Féin for its salvation.'[2] The influenza pandemic had a curious synchronicity with developments in struggle between the state and nationalists, as this chapter teases out. It dealt a useful hand to the Sinn Féin network of professional and citizen propagandists, who managed to adapt the disease as a political tool, in both a deliberate and subliminal way.

There were essentially three strands to the influence of Spanish influenza on the independence movement; the purpose of this chapter is to explore them. Each strand provided material which the advanced nationalists could work into their anti-Government propaganda: influenza among cultural and political nationalists within communities, the treatment received by DORA political prisoners suffering from influenza in Belfast jail, and the threat posed by influenza to leading members of Sinn Féin and others interned in Great Britain under alleged suspicion of involvement in the so-called 'German' plot. Many of the internees stood in the December 1918 general election, which added a further dimension to the interest in their detention and well-being, particularly within their constituencies. Some sent speeches to be read at the pre-election rallies, often mentioning the conditions and unjust nature of their detention, and the health of the prisoners.

Surveying regional newspapers with nationalist sympathies shows that they carried, alongside stories illustrating the Government's ineptitude in dealing with the influenza crisis, extensive obituaries and coverage of the funerals of Sinn Féin activists who died from the influenza. They used the opportunity provided by the epidemic to eulogise the victims and establish their credentials as Fíor-Ghaels, or true Irish patriots. The attendance at their funerals, sometimes estimated at several thousand, was a gauge of popular support for their ideals. A typical example was the death report and obituary of James Corrigan, aged twenty-seven, who was a teacher in Birr Co. Offaly. The *Midland Tribune* states his Fíor Ghael qualifications. He taught Irish, was secretary of Offaly Gaelic Athletic Association, and of South Offaly Gaelic League, was a member of Sinn Féin and the Irish Volunteers, captain of a championship winning Offaly hurling team and possessed of such a talent for organisation that even at a young age he had been the mainspring for athletic activity in the county, an 'assiduous reviver of the native tongue', and an officer of the Irish Volunteers who was a strict disciplinarian and ardent Catholic. He was a veritable all-round Fíor Ghael, as his obituary proclaims:[3]

> His mind was filled with the purest and loftiest ideals emanating from a soul burning with patriotism, and faithfully irradiating the piercing light which constitutes Irish nationality. He fully realized that national liberty was not a toy to be bartered away, but an ideal to be purchased only by wading through the deepest suffering and pain.

By establishing the cultural and political nationalism of the influenza victims in their obituaries and at their funerals, propagandists were effectively harnessing their deaths to the Irish patriot funerary tradition. The burials of nineteenth-century parliamentarians Daniel O'Connell and Charles Stewart Parnell were renowned for their grandeur and popular support, while Patrick Pearse's stirring oratory at the stage-managed 1915 funeral of the Fenian Jeremiah O'Donovan Rossa had invested the sentimental tradition with real political impetus, seizing an opportunity to display the growing strength of the Irish Volunteers.[4] So much so, that in 1916, General Maxwell feared that 'Irish sentimentality' would turn the graves of the executed leaders of the Rising 'into martyr's shrines' and ordered that the corpses be buried with discreet haste in quicklime in a mass grave at the military cemetery in Arbour Hill in Dublin, rather than in what had become the traditional burial ground for the nationalist dead at Glasnevin Cemetery.[5] Part of the power of the patriot funeral came from the place of the funeral in Irish society in general. Thomas J. Brophy has argued that because mourning practices were such an important feature of community life, nationalist obsequies' organisers played upon the people's emotions and customs as much or more than their political inclinations: 'They gained easy access to the public consciousness and lodged their message into the collective memory.'[6] Framing the deaths of Irish nationalists to influence the opinions of the living against the Government was something of an art form by 1918. Even if the victims had died from a global pandemic that was completely outside the control of the British or any other government, the propaganda potential in pre-election months was too useful to ignore.

Influenza among DORA prisoners in Ireland

Influenza was used to highlight perceptions of mistreatment of Sinn Féin DORA prisoners in Belfast jail in a long-running and very public squabble between the Irish Chief Secretary, Edward Shortt, the General Prisons Board for Ireland, the prisoners and their lawyers. This dispute was perceived by the GPB and others as being a major threat to prison security, and not only in Belfast. Convicted Sinn Féin prisoners in Cork, Galway, Limerick, Derry, Mountjoy and Waterford, who had been granted 'ameliorations', were awaiting transfer to a special section of the prison in Belfast, where it was proposed to keep them under conditions for well-behaved internees. The move was suspended indefinitely when flu broke out among DORA prisoners in Belfast jail; prison authorities, fearful that the suspension would lead to some sort of an attack on the prisons involved, mounted extra guards on those prisons.[7] All of this was informed by a serious disturbance among the republican prisoners with special ameliorations in June 1918.[8] As conditions in Belfast deteriorated, informed observers warned that if blood were to be spilt in Belfast prison, it would have a domino effect in other parts of the country as the situation was being closely watched.[9]

By 25 October, the GPB felt it expedient to report to the Under-Secretary, James MacMahon, that there had been a serious outbreak of influenza in the jail with eighty of the DORA prisoners affected. The GPB's medical member, Dr MacCormack, was on his way to Belfast to confer with the prison's medical officer about how to deal with the outbreak.[10] The row really began when a solicitor for the prisoners, Mr McGinn, wrote to Chief Secretary Edward Shortt, seeking the admission of three named doctors to treat Sinn Féin prisoners in Belfast prison suffering from influenza.[11] His letter had scarcely arrived on 28 October 1918 when a series of telegrams from various parties involved in the Sinn Féin propaganda operations barraged the Chief Secretary's office, as the condition of the prisoners worsened. They claimed that 111 political prisoners were down with the flu. Their conditions, they alleged, were disgraceful: the men were locked in their cells with only dry bread and tea for food, were sleeping on floors with poor quality bedding and were not receiving sufficient medical treatment. They had no nurses or hospital accommodation, and wanted to have doctors admitted whom they could trust to care for them.[12] These allegations were published in several newspapers.

The prison governor, William Barrows, reported by telephone to the GPB on 28 October that there were 111 DORA prisoners sick with influenza, along with fourteen officers, including two clerks. He had employed eleven temporary warders; the great number of sick was placing a great strain on the officers left on duty, as they had to provide nursing day and night. He asked that three ordinary warders be sent at once to help, as the prison needed more trained warders; the board seconded three warders from other prisons on 29 October.[13]

DORA prisoner Micéal Costello's letter of 5 November 1918 to his wife Teresa Costello, Round Tower Road, Clondalkin, was suppressed by Governor Barrows, as he said it contained inaccurate information about the epidemic. It appears, however, to have been well grounded in fact:

My dear Cissie,

Just a few lines to let you know that the 'flu' is raging here at its height. Sixteen patients are gone to outside hospitals I am so far keeping clear of it. It is a very dangerous form of sickness nose-bleeding, terrible sweats, weakness, pain in the chest, horrible coughs, getting better and then getting worse. My God, you would pity the men in the cells beads of sweat standing out on their faces. You can imagine what it would be in a home but in a prison cell, it is absolute murder. No man is sent outside unless he is dangerously ill, that is when he has developed pneumonia. We are getting fairly well treated now but there are 70 in the cells yet. They should be sent to a proper hospital. There are plenty of beds to be had in Lisburn Road, that is the Union Hospital in Belfast. I found Murphy lying on the floor one morning at 7 am and I found (another prisoner) bleeding to death, the latter is the worst case of the lot outside now. There are some bad cases here yet some men don't get any medicine on some days unless our own fellows find that he has not got it. The lads very much neglected in the early stages of the flu. There is a night and day nurse here for the last few days, they are trying to kill us with kindness now. I hope there will be no casualties and please God there won't be. Tell all that I was asking for them. Hoping yourself, Maureen, Kit and Masey are well. Remain your loving husband Micéal.[14]

More details of prison conditions during the epidemic came from prisoner Mícéal Stapleton in a letter addressed to his sister Josie Stapleton, Main Street, Kilcock, Co. Kildare (the letter is simply dated Wednesday, but the correspondence number suggests it was written in early November 1918). Again, it was suppressed by Captain Barrows who claimed it included improper comments about the treatment of prisoners:

> The number of patients here is very considerable. Today there are between 120 and 130 down – some of whom have been removed to the Mater hospital, having developed pneumonia. I don't know how many of them have been removed – but I am sure that there are six at least. Then, seventeen are in the prison hospital, and the remaining number – 107 – are in their cells. Of course the work upon those who have been spared so far is somewhat strenuous; but we are most happy to be able to do something for our suffering fellow-prisoners. It is a glaring piece of injustice that no trained nurses have been requisitioned to attend properly to our poor suffering comrades. Nursing is a profession which we cannot be expected to know. So far TG none of my comrades nor I have been stricken. Undoubtedly, the danger is great … it is, to my mind, an absurd thing to call it 'flu' or 'influenza' for it is in reality a fever of a very dangerous kind … As far as possible, we should all guard against panic; for that in itself, leaves us all liable to fall victim. We should remain, calm, cool and confident. Although we have seen, and have helped to remove some of our comrades on stretchers, we have not become panic-stricken. The stretcher is as familiar to us now as is the prison 'tray' … Now, don't feel anxious about me I am remaining in very best health and hope to remain so until PG I am at liberty to see you all again. Your loving brother Mícéal.[15]

The Sinn Féin prisoners conducted a series of protests in order to gain proper care for their colleagues who were ill with influenza. The General Prisons Board for Ireland refused to permit the prisoners to receive private medical attention, instead directing the prison governor to improve the conditions under which the prisoners were kept during the epidemic; they received extra medical and nursing care and proper beds, bedding and mattresses. Ill prisoners were permitted to have cell doors open, and were given a special diet. The epidemic and the ensuing relaxation in the prison regime caused considerable strain on the prison staff; most of them were middle-aged, whereas the prisoners were generally younger. With the new open-cell-door policy, the staff felt under threat from prisoners who could now potentially arm themselves with bedposts; according to a GPB inspector's report in late November, eighteen of the staff were ill with influenza and absent and the chief warder had 'lost his reason' from the strain.[16] Barrows' communications with the GPB throughout November and December documented his fears about the possibility of violence breaking out in the prison among the special prisoners when the relaxation of rules necessitated by the influenza outbreak eventually had to be reversed. His letter to the Board on 7 November 1918, advising that some of the prisoners were now recovered, and were walking around the yard but still complaining of pains and aches, warned:

> If I enforce the rules it will be looked upon as oppression and will probably be exaggerated in the press and correspondence, but under existing conditions convalescent patients can and do exchange visits with each other in the different wards at all hours up to 12 midnight, and proper supervision is difficult to manage, there are still a number of prisoners who are really sick, and it would not in my opinion be advisable to take extreme measures just now.

The chairman of the GPB, Max Green, and other board members agreed that Barrows should take a cautious approach. Reporting to Under-Secretary MacMahon, Green wrote that there was a great spirit of unrest among the special prisoners in Belfast, and that the Board had been informed that a similar spirit of unrest was among other special prisoners also, and that as the prison warders were not fit to deal with trouble, they might be supplemented by a special military guard.

When the epidemic appeared to have ended in December 1918, the Board was considering the reinstigation of the pre-epidemic regime. The prisoners used the opportunity to riot, using parts of the new beds as missiles: they conducted a rooftop protest, and later blockaded themselves into a section of the prison.[17] The pressure took its toll on the governor, Captain Barrows, who took suddenly ill with an acute attack of cardiac vertigo on 30 December 1918, and was replaced by the governor of Maryborough Prison, Horatio Chippindall.[18]

The Belfast prisoners' dispute continued into the spring of 1919, with another outbreak of influenza occurring in the prison in March.[19] The alleged mistreatment of the ill prisoners by Belfast prison authorities and their political masters was well publicised by the organisation. Sinn Féin had capitalised on the row, attracting public attention to the prisoners' plight. Ultimately, no Sinn Féin prisoner in Belfast jail died from influenza, perhaps as a result of ameliorations in their treatment enforced by the publicity, which clearly influenced the authorities.

Influenza and the 'German' plot internees

Perhaps the more interesting influence of Spanish influenza on nationalist politics was in relation to the so-called 'German' plot. In early March 1918, a German spring offensive on the Western Front compelled the British Government to consider extending conscription to Ireland; on the face of it, Ireland could provide a relatively untapped source of manpower for the war effort. Irish Chief Secretary Henry Duke warned that he might as well conscript Germans as Irishmen. Others advised that introducing conscription to Ireland would lead to chaos.[20] David Lloyd George, the British Prime Minister, introduced a military conscription bill on 9 April. He delayed its application to Ireland, but the immediate response was to unify the somewhat disjointed broad spectrum of Irish nationalists into a national conscription resistance campaign.[21] Within days, it was announced that a nationalist, Joe Dowling, had been arrested following his landing by a German submarine on the Clare coast. British intelligence started to investigate an alleged plot by the Germans to provide an expeditionary force to support another nationalist rising.

Popular support for the anti-conscription movement escalated rapidly. Public meetings held in Dublin and around the country drew large crowds. Duke was highly agitated, as William Murphy notes, and warned the Cabinet that the Irish situation was critical. On the basis of the chief secretary's advice, the regulations enacting DORA were amended on 20 April to allow interment if individuals acted 'in a manner prejudicial to the public safety of the realm'.[22] On 5 May 1918, the government replaced Chief Secretary Duke and Lord Lieutenant Lord Wimborne with an Irish executive who more fully supported their intent to enforce conscription. They wanted a team who would play hard ball with the anti-conscription movement, an increasingly popular broad

alignment of nationalists from many organisations. Edward Shortt
became chief secretary and Sir John French became lord lieutenant. The new executive rounded up prominent anti-conscription
campaigners under alleged suspicion of collusion with Germany: it
was perhaps no coincidence that DORR 14B permitted the detention of individuals with 'hostile origin or association'.[23] Initially,
sixty-nine people were arrested on the night of 17 May 1918, and
more were arrested in the following days and months; many of
these were transported to Britain where they were interned
without charge.[24] The internees included three women who each
had an almost iconic status in Irish society: Cumann na mBan
president Constance Markievicz, an aristocrat whose nationalist
credentials had been forged by the roles she played both in the
1913 Lockout and in the 1916 rising, poet W.B. Yeats' muse and
founder of Inghinidhe na hÉireann Maud Gonne McBride, and
Kathleen Clarke, who had nationalist credentials in her own right
as a vice-president of Cumann na mBan and a member of Sinn
Féin's executive, but also had the added cachet of being the widow
of executed 1916 leader Thomas Clarke: the 1916 rebellion signa-
tories, through their hasty post-rebellion executions were regarded
as national martyrs in Ireland. Clarke's arrest caused a particular
outcry, as her three small sons, who had already lost their father,
were now left temporarily motherless, and she was known to be in
frail health. The women were sent to Holloway jail, in Islington.
The men detained included Arthur Griffith and Eamon de Valera,
and several journalists who worked on propaganda, including
Willie Brennan Whitmore and Robert Brennan. They went to Usk,
Birmingham, Gloucester, Durham, Lincoln and Reading prisons.

Irish history is peppered with stories of perceived British injustice
towards Ireland's nationalist politicians. The 'German' plot case quickly
became one of these perceived injustices; even Lord Wimborne
suggested that evidence in support of the plot was flimsy. Nationalists
portrayed it as yet another example of British hypocrisy. From their
perspective, Britain was fighting in a war to protect the 'freedom of
small nations', whereas on the domestic front it had interned Irish political activists seeking the right to self-determination to become one
of those small nations that Britain claimed to defend.[25] The 'German'
plot became a coup not for the perceived oppressor but the perceived
oppressed, as public opinion was swiftly persuaded by pro-nationalist

propaganda carefully placed in the news pages. As 'Johanna' from Westport wrote to the interned P. Sugrue on 24 November 1918:

> You are more of a power in Irish affairs than if you were out. We all love the 'felons of our land.' You know now that the election fight is here we must arouse the best feelings and sympathies of the nation, and the silence of Sinn Féin Leaders because enforced is more effective than any amount of ability from the platform.[26]

Jail was not a new experience for many of the internees. William Murphy argued that prisoners and their supporters were very much aware of the potential propaganda dividend that political prisoners and their supporters could extract: 'That many of the significant figures in Dáil Éireann's, Sinn Féin's, and the Irish Volunteers' publicity and propaganda departments (e.g. Desmond FitzGerald, Frank Gallagher, Piaras Beaslaí and Arthur Griffith) had themselves been prisoners ideally equipped them for this task.'[27]

After an initial settling-in period, as terms and conditions were negotiated between the prisoners and the prison authorities and the Home Office, terms were relatively relaxed, with the men and women being treated as civil detainees, although assigned to a prison rather than a camp.[28] Their correspondence was supposed to be strictly monitored by a postal censor, and all communications from the internees carried to the press were required to be submitted to the press censor. Despite these instructions, news occasionally managed to appear in the newspapers and the press censor would administer a rebuke to the newspaper editors.[29]

The first wave of influenza broke out in mid-June, shortly after the round-up. Three of the internees were medical doctors, Richard Hayes, Bryan Cusack and H. Russell McNabb. There were repeated appeals in the Dublin and regional newspapers for the release of the three to tend to influenza patients during the crisis, from several BOGs and Dublin Corporation meetings.[30] There were also appeals for Kathleen Lynn, who had evaded detention, although she had been visiting Tommy and Geraldine Dillon when Tommy Dillon was arrested, to come off 'the run'. After hearing at a Sinn Féin standing committee meeting that the entire executive was to be arrested, she called in on the way home. In her diary, on that evening, she entered: 'G men came while Dr D. and I were at the door. He was taken. I walked out and off.' The next day, Saturday 18 May she noted: 'Almost whole executive arrested and deported. myself "on the run".' The following day the diary notes: 'Whit Sunday. German plot "discovered" by French. No one believes it.'[31] Following negotiations mediated by the Lord Mayor of Dublin Laurence O'Neill, Lynn was arrested early in the morning of 31 October, brought to Rathmines police station and then to Arbour Hill, where the deportation order was cancelled on the proviso that she tend to the ill and abstained from politics.[32]

The influenza epidemic, unpredictable and life-threatening as it was, naturally caused extra anxiety for families separated as a result of the 'German' plot. Sinn Féin sympathisers and the families of internees wrote to newspapers and to the prisoners of their concerns that the prisoners (many of whom were in poor health from previous incarcerations) would not cope well if the influenza epidemic were to arrive in their prisons.[33] Equally, those inside fretted about the health of loved ones at home; the postal censor remarked that some of the prisoners' letters home were showing considerable depression about the ravages of the influenza epidemic in Ireland.[34] The correspondence both in and out of prison and memoirs show that the nationalist leadership and their families had close friendships: Kathleen Lynn's terse diary entries show frequent worries about Kathleen Clarke, Maud Gonne and the Dillons; ironically, Clarke caught flu when she was released from jail in February 1919, and was treated by Lynn. Gonne was released from Holloway in November 1918 and ordered to stay near a sanatorium in Ipswich until further order.[35] Markievicz was released in March 1919.

Geraldine Dillon, Tommy's wife, who was also the daughter of another internee Count George Noble Plunkett, gave birth to their second daughter Blánaid on 26 May 1918. In the middle of a hot June, the mother and her two infant daughters caught the Spanish influenza. Their first carer fell ill with flu herself. A chance call by a relative who found the household in a bad way led to the procuring of a nurse for the family. Dillon recalled: 'I remember trying to nurse poor Bláth, who was a month old and had got it badly with a temperature of 104 degrees. I would wake up to find myself waking her up by singing her to sleep in a loud voice.'[36] In mid-October, one of the internees, Offaly county councillor Thomas M. Russell, Ballyduff House, Tullamore, was temporarily released from Birmingham, when all four of his children were threatened with death by influenza. Before he arrived, his eldest son Cecil, aged ten, had lapsed into a coma and only survived his father's arrival by a few hours. The boy died on Wednesday 16 October.[37] Russell was not required to return to jail, and the chief secretary made an order of revocation in his case on 2 December 1918.[38]

Kathleen Clarke revealed some of this fear surrounding the disease in her autobiography:

> Then we read of the terrible epidemic of 'flu raging all over England and Ireland. The newspapers were full of it. In a letter from home I got news that some members of the family were already down with it, and for weeks after that there was no letter. I was sick with anxiety. What was wrong that I had no letters from home? Were they all dead? At the end of five weeks I got a big bunch of letters. They had been held up in the Censor's Office. I wondered if the Censor knew what suffering he had caused me ... the news was good. The family were neither dying nor dead, though some of them had had the flu. The think the anxiety made whatever was wrong with my heart worse, as the attacks became more frequent, accompanied by sharp pain. Still, I would not consult the doctor.

Gonne and Markievicz frequently expressed concern in their letters about Clarke's health. Gonne had been determined to go on hunger strike, but was put off the idea when Clarke and Markievicz declared that they would join her on it. Gonne said in her witness statement: 'I knew it would kill Kathleen and I tried to dissuade her, but they were determined, so I gave up on that occasion.'[39] Markievicz wrote to Hanna Sheehy Skeffington in October 1918:

> We are very anxious about Mrs. C[larke]. No matter how strong her spirit it is clear that her health suffers gravely and that is not surprising. And as for Mrs. [Gonne] McBride, I think lung trouble is always a treacherous malady, and apt to recur when the condition of health is low.[40]

Both Clarke and Gonne found Markievicz's concern somewhat overbearing, and resented her expressing fears in her letters that might alarm their families. The three were uncomfortable companions, constantly complaining about each other and at the same time concerned about each other, and sharing a spirit of adventure.[41] Markievicz did not share the belief – or follow the propaganda narrative – that prison was a dangerous place to be in during the pandemic, unlike Gonne who had stressed the awfulness of the conditions, that the Holloway cells were small. Ever pragmatic, Markievicz wrote to Mrs Wyse Power that in Holloway – where she, Maud Gonne and Kathleen Clarke were being detained – they were safer from flu than outside, and that there was no cause for alarm: the conditions under which they were being held were not conducive towards making them ill. Their cells had, she said, large windows and hot pipes, and they had been provided with 'quite decent' winter clothes.[42] Maud Gonne in her Bureau of Military History witness statement pointed out, it might be said gleefully, how the three discovered by chance that these very cells which Markievicz praised were in fact the cells normally reserved for prisoners suffering from syphilis. They found out when Markievicz grabbed a rather larger towel than the small one she had been given from a pile on her way into the washroom, and one of the warders shouted at her to stop: 'Don't you know that this is the syphilis wing and that your linen is washed apart?'[43]

In late November, several of the internees in Usk jail caught the flu, and at first were nursed by their colleagues, and had no medical care as the prison doctor was away at war. George Lyons, who had been released because of ill health in January 1919, told the *Irish Independent* that Coleman and the Gorey journalist Willie Brennan Whitmore came down with flu on 30 November. 'Up to this time', said Mr Lyons, 'the nursing was being done by ourselves, and we were naturally contracting the disease, delicate men stopping up at night to attend to their comrades'. On 1 December, a resident doctor was provided, and the following day the invalids were removed to new hospital wards. On 6 December, a nurse came to assist the medical officer. Coleman died on 9 December; his emotional comrades carried his corpse late at night, in a downpour of rain, over two prison yards to their wing of the prison. Lyons added that the condition of two other prisoners, Whitmore and Donovan, was in January still causing anxiety.[44]

Coleman (who was already a hero because of his part in the 1916 rebellion and in the hunger strike in which Thomas Ashe died in 1917) had now become a martyr by dying from influenza. His timing could not have been more effective for the cause of Sinn Féin, who claimed his death as a murder in prison: the general election was to

be held on 14 December.[45]. Sinn Féin moved swiftly to capitalise on
the present handed to them by fate. Pro-nationalist newspapers gave
columns of coverage to the tragic circumstances of the Swords man's
death. A party advertisement on the front page of the leading daily
newspaper, the *Irish Independent*, claimed that Coleman had joined
the ranks of martyrs who had died for Ireland, as the last of a long
list extending from High King Brian Boru's death at the Battle of
Clontarf in 1014 (see Figure 14).[46]

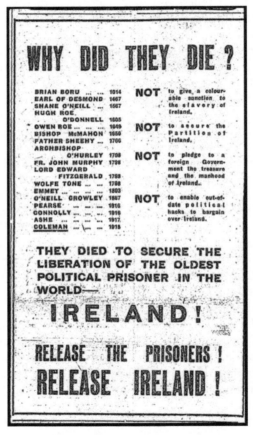

Figure 17 'Why did they die?' advertisement, front page, *Irish Independent*,
12 December 1918, adds influenza victim Richard Coleman to a list of Irish
political martyrs.

The postal censor noted that Coleman's death gave rise to a certain amount of hostile criticism in prison correspondence. Letters both to and from Ireland showed that efforts were being made to exploit it as a further instance of the perceived British inhumanity towards the Irish. The censor listed extracts which exemplified the attitude adopted by the internees and their relatives:

J O'REILLY TO MRS O'REILLY 10.12.18: 'Poor Dick Coleman ... he had been hunted and persecuted more than any I know of and he died in Usk prison the victim of the arch-hypocrite that mouths about humanity and the 'rights of small nationalities'. Oh God, how long must our people suffer. We sent him home to Ireland yesterday evening after being kept here from Monday to convenience the coroner who went through an obviously rehearsed farce called an inquest.'

FROM MRS MELLOWS, DUBLIN, 12.12.18: 'I am greatly upset to hear of poor Coleman's death and of his having gone to his long-earned rest ... that most human of governments can torture him no longer. He has now joined that noble band of Irish martyrs in Heaven.'[47]

Much of the prison correspondence openly blamed the British authorities for Coleman's death rather than attributing his demise to the chance contracting of an infectious epidemic disease. A letter to Bernard Fallon from Bridget O'Flanagan directs the blame:

Although the authorities say his death was caused by the flu, that is not taking the responsibility off them. Thomas Ashe was murdered and forcibly fed – poor Coleman was left to die in the want of proper treatment in those filthy cells, and his brother at the door, and when poor Richard was gone he was admitted. Oh the savages! But however, he died for a good cause, for the love of his country. What all our brave boys are ready to do ... as I say often, the more they arrest, and what is more, the more they murder, the stronger we are ... But who knows what may turn up. But perhaps they want to kill more of you with the flu by the way.[48]

C.F. Stafford in Drumcondra wrote to Kathleen Clarke in Holloway:

I expect you heard they finished Dick Coleman RIP in Usk jail last Monday ... All Ireland mourns him today ... He was murdered just as they murdered Thomas Ashe only in a different manner.

Eamon de Valera wrote to his wife Sinéad the previous day:

> Poor Dick Coleman has I see gone to join his comrades on the other side. They are going one by one but I know no greater consolation they could have than that they are being granted – their deaths are fresh embers to the flames which they lovingly tended during life. Fingal has contributed more than its share. May god grant Ireland no end of sons like brave gentle Dick.[49]

In a letter on 13 December 1918, M. Spillane's mother mentioned the heightened tensions that the families of those still interned must have been feeling:

> We are anxious particularly on account of the sad occurrence at Usk. Is it not dreadful, a young fellow dying in an English prison so far from home and friends? I daresay if he had been at home he would be well nourished and cared for. He would be alive and well today, but he hadn't much chance to pull through in a cold damp cell.[50]

Frank Gallagher, who was working for the interned Sinn Féin Director of Publicity Robert Brennan at the time, evaluated Coleman's death from the perspective of its use as propaganda:

> He was but 27 years of age; he was handsome. It was as if a goodly knight had fallen in a crusade. The people's tears came quickly for him. The inquest disclosed the utter neglect of the sick in Usk prison, where there was not even a trained nurse … The disclosure horrified all who had men in prison … The morning after the Coleman inquest canvassers sought out those still doubtful and put straight questions to them. How could any but the heartless stand aside now? All over Ireland that night the 'Ds'(canvas tallies for 'doubtful', F for 'for' and A for 'against') were being rubbed out.[51]

Coleman's body was brought back to Dublin on 13 December, arriving from Kingstown port into Westland Row railway station where his family and a crowd of a thousand people, including Mrs Pearse, the mother of the executed 1916 rebellion hero, Patrick, the newspapers reported; the coffin was carried on the shoulders of Volunteers into St Andrew's Church next door, pending burial in Glasnevin Cemetery on the day after the election.[52] That evening, the final election rally was held in Dublin's O'Connell Street, with Sinn Féin's banners and posters newly draped with black mourning ribbons. Frank Gallagher described the scene, with each of the city constituencies was represented by its own speakers in its wagonette: 'Down the whole length of the great thoroughfare the nine city meetings were held and over each flew a tricolour with a black cross on every one for Dick Coleman. Thousands wore the enamel badges with their candidate's photograph, draped now in crêpe.' The mourning colours were for Coleman, but perhaps also were resounding of the losses represented by the 1916 rebellion backdrop of O'Connell Street, and the leading players in the rally, as Gallagher indicates: 'Mrs. Pearse presided at the main meeting; Mrs. Ceannt and others of the 1916 women presided at others.'[53] In her diaries, Kathleen Lynn refers to it as 'the memorable day before the poll, a wonderful evening in O'Connell Street. M (her companion Madeleine Ffrench Mullen) and I got stand room on a brake and heard K. Flanagan. The flags, banners and torches were a sight to see. A lovely moonlit night.'[54]

On election day itself, the *Evening Herald* carried detailed instructions from the Sinn Féin headquarters at 6 Harcourt Street, telling a long list of groups, including Coleman's fellow employees at the New Ireland Assurance Society, the Irish Volunteers, Cumann na mBan and the Irish Women's Franchise League what role they were to play in the funeral procession and the path it would take through the city. The affiliated bodies of the trades council, representing 25,000 workers, had been instructed to attend the funeral in full force. This level of stage management indicates that the organisation was clearly keen to exploit the opportunity of Coleman's funeral to make an impression on the Government and on the electorate.[55] He would have the classic patriot funeral, in the tradition of Parnell, with the streets of the second city in the Union as a backdrop. But stage management alone did not explain the 15,000 people who turned out in a rain-stricken Dublin in his honour, Séan McConville has argued. The hearse was led through the streets by 60 Volunteers and 50 priests, and followed by a long line of carriages, including Lord Mayor O'Neill, and several hundred more Volunteers in formation.[56]

In the background, the Home Office and the Irish Office were continually corresponding on issues concerning the prisoners. After Coleman died in Usk jail, C.A. Hunt from the Home Office told S.M. Power in the Irish Office:

Dear Power,

We have received the following telegram: 'Irish trained nurses to leave for English prisons nurse Irish prisoners stricken with influenza. Wire necessary permits, Sheehan Secretary Sinn Féin, 6 Harcourt St,

Dublin'. (We) should be glad to know what reply the chief secretary wishes sent. I am informed by the prison commissioners that they have made all necessary provision and that nurses are not required, and as a matter of fact the epidemic at Usk is abating and the worst is over,

Yours sincerely
C.A. Hunt.[57]

A handwritten note on this letter from Hunt instructed that a response should be sent saying that all necessary provision had been made and that nurses were therefore not required.

When the election results came in, Sinn Féin had a resounding victory in the election, winning seventy-three seats. In Dublin, they had expected to take nine of the eleven seats, and took ten, with Desmond FitzGerald taking the tenth, for which Gallagher pays tribute to the 'inexhaustible energy' of his wife Mabel who managed his campaign while Desmond was still interned.[58] P.S. O'Hegarty believed the vote was reactionary: 'The victory of Christmas 1918 was not a victory of conviction, but of emotion. It was a victory occasioned less by any sudden achievement by the majority of a belief in Ireland a nation than by the sudden reaction against various acts of English tyranny.'[59] Whether or not Coleman's death and the way he was presented to the electorate as a martyr for the cause were, in fact, effective in increasing the vote for Sinn Féin is open to speculation. Robert Brennan, Sinn Féin director of publicity and also director of elections until his internment in Gloucester three weeks before the election, claimed that he had predicted the number of seats several weeks before, indicating that Coleman's death made little impact on the vote. But there may have been some professional jealousy of his subordinate at the time, Frank Gallagher, who wrote about it having a deep impact on the electorate.[60] In a pamphlet published after the release of the prisoners in 1919, Sinn Féin claimed that Coleman's death was murder.[61]

In another irony of the epidemic, at the time when prisoners at Gloucester jail were hit by a severe bout of influenza in the third wave in mid-February, their jailer-in-chief Lord French was also confined to bed with the disease. French's absence from official engagements was explained in the *Irish Times* on 11 February 1919 to be a result of his suffering from bronchitis following influenza. He returned to the Vice-Regal Lodge two months later, but some commentators observed that the flu and subsequent bronchitis and pneumonia permanently reduced the vitality of a man who had previously been known for his energy.[62]

At the end of February, more political prisoners – this time at Gloucester and Durham – were reported to be suffering from the flu. At the beginning of March five of the eleven political prisoners in Durham jail were ill, while Arthur Griffith sent a message that relatives of the ten men in Gloucester jail, who were suffering from influenza, should not be alarmed.[63] Frank Drohan, who had been one of those nursing the influenza patients in Usk jail when Dick Coleman died, caught the flu himself in Gloucester:

> I remember the nurse coming around to check my temperature and pulse and I noticed her making an involuntary exclamation when she noticed the temperature and whilst she was writing on the chart. I said to the lads beside me, 'I must be bad'. I climbed up to have a look at the chart and saw that it registered 104. I was in a kind of trance for about three days, delirium I suppose. I remember I was going through halls and all kinds of grand places during that time.[64]

Darrell Figgis, who was home on parole, told an *Irish Independent* reporter that many of the prisoners were weakened by their long confinement; the latest victims had seemed to him to be the fittest of all and he feared for the others. They were fed the same food as the convicts, and their cells were like icehouses.[65] Figgis had a tendency to exaggerate, but the situation was bad, nonetheless. Robert Brennan recalled that a warder, who seemed very much afraid of catching the flu, told him that it had reached Gloucester, and that people were dying like flies. To Brennan's surprise, the warder himself died during that night from influenza. The authorities acted prudently, by sending the seriously ill prisoners to nursing homes. Brennan wrote that the prison stank of plague. 'By the doctor's order, we were allowed to exercise in a larger ground where we could play rounders and we were served with doses of a particularly potent tonic each evening just before lock-up time.' The flu occasionally gave a much-needed opportunity for light relief. J.K. O'Reilly protested that the doctor had prescribed him whiskey instead of tonic, and at Arthur Griffith's instigation the internees refused to go back to their cells at bedtime until he got the prescribed medicine, whiskey. After a stand-off with the chief warder, the governor was called. Under pressure and repeated teasing from Griffith, he brought a bottle of whiskey. The prisoners gleefully recognised this as a confiscated bottle of Dunville's whiskey from Belfast which had been sent to Sean MacEntee at Christmas. 'Lads, go get your mugs', said McEntee. Brennan recounted that the whiskey was shared, and it was a great night as many of the internees were teetotallers.[66]

Some of the prisoners' families came to nurse them and found conditions very inadequate, even though the authorities had removed them to Beaufort Buildings Spa, a private nursing home in Gloucester.[67] Geraldine Plunkett Dillon recalled arriving at a nursing home where there were twenty men in one room and eight in another, 'closely packed'; her husband Tommy was one of the most ill. All the staff had flu. She reported that Pierce McCan had become violent with the fever, a not unusual side effect. McCan, scion of wealthy farming stock and newly elected MP for Tipperary East, got pneumonia and was isolated from the rest of the patients.[68] Robert Brennan, newly released from Gloucester, told an *Irish Independent* reporter:

> Much to the astonishment of us all we were told that Mr McCan's condition had grown worse. He was one of the strongest men in the prison, and excelled in games of handball, rounders, etc. but the confinement told upon him much more than on others because he was used to outdoor life and exercise.

McCan had called into Brennan's cell to discuss his concerns about the flu, as some of the warders were off sick. He had quizzed the prison doctor about the potential of the flu to kill if it infected the prisoners. The doctor told him that it was quite possible that it would, so McCan asked if any precautions were being taken, and subsequently complained that nothing was being done to prevent the spread of the epidemic among the prisoners. Brennan remarked: 'He seemed to be afraid of the disease, apparently on account of his system being run down.'

The Government, at last becoming wary of the expected adverse publicity if another prisoner died, made a decision to release the prisoners. Ian Macpherson, who had replaced Shortt as chief secretary since January, began issuing staggered release orders to evade the impact that a mass release would have made. On 6 March, as the authorities were beginning to sign orders for a release of the prisoners, Pierce McCan, aged thirty-five, died. His loss was a major shock – the intellectual and pious McCan was renowned for his athleticism and heroism. His robust pre-incarceration health was in no doubt, given that he had cycled long distances to anti-conscription rallies the previous year. McCan taught French in the prison, and sang and played the flute. He was, Robert Brennan said, very popular with all the prisoners. He was a handsome hero and popular with women, as the letters in his National Library of Ireland collection testify. The report of his death in the *Irish Independent* described him as the third member of Sinn Féin to die in custody (the others being Coleman and Thomas Ashe, who had died while on hunger strike in 1917), president of the East Tipperary Sinn Féin Executive and prominent in the Irish language movement: 'A gentleman of magnificent physique, he was one of the most daring riders with the east Tipperary Hunt.'[69] The circumstances and timing of McCan's death once again played straight into the welcoming hands of the Sinn Féin propaganda machine. Although the release orders had been issued before his death, the public perception was that he had died in captivity, forcing the Government to release the rest.

The funeral Sinn Féin orchestrated for McCan surpassed even the excesses of that of Coleman: 10,000 people were reported to have followed the hearse to the Pro-cathedral in Dublin, before another imposing procession through crowd-lined streets to Kingsbridge station, with members of Dáil Éireann marching behind the hearse. His corpse was taken by train to Thurles for burial, in a van draped with an enormous Sinn Féin flag; crowds stood on platforms of stations along the way. Archbishop Harty and sixteen other priests conducted the service in Thurles. The removal to the burial ground at his family home was again an enormous affair, even by the standards of Sinn Féin funerals, with forty-three priests at the graveside. Every funeral orator and every dignitary issuing a public statement used the opportunity to lay the blame for the death of yet another gallant young Fíor Ghael at the hands of the Government, which detained him without trial and refused to release him when the flu presented a dangerous threat to his health.

A *Tipperary Star* journalist eulogised him in hagiographical terms, in a special black-bordered funeral edition: 'Our latest hero-martyr whose stainless, sinless soul has freed itself, and his great fearless spirit has gone forth amid a nation's grief and sorrow. Worthy indeed to be linked with Ashe and Coleman.'[70] The timing of and the publicity about Richard Coleman's death in the days immediately preceding the general election probably consolidated an already strong Sinn Féin vote. Sinn Féin's orchestration of his funeral through the streets of Dublin the day after the general election was intended as a show of force as well as a show of mourning. Pierce McCan's death enabled Sinn Féin's propagandists to promulgate their message of the unjust treatment Irish nationalists received at the hands of the British Government, in order to create the illusion that his death had shamed the Government into releasing the rest of the prisoners, and to use his enormous funeral as a show of force.[71]

Sinn Féin capitalised on the deaths of Coleman and McCan, although neither victim held pivotal roles within the organisation. Arthur Griffith, on the other hand, did. He caught flu, but against all the prevailing advice, insisted on fighting it on his feet. Bob Brennan, in his autobiography, *Allegiance*, described Griffith's tussle with Spanish influenza:

> One morning, while the flu raged, when our numbers had been reduced by one-half, AG did not turn up for breakfast. I went to his cell and found him half awake. One glance showed me he had it. 'How are you feeling' 'I'm alright', he said, starting to get up. 'Stay where you are, I said. I'll bring your breakfast.' 'No, I'm getting up', he said. My eye caught the tonic bottle the orderly had left the night before. It was empty. 'What happened this?' I asked. 'I drank it last night.' 'All of it?' Yes.' 'You were to take only three tablespoons a day.' 'Well, if a spoonful is good, a bottle is better', he said, trying to grin. 'That's the stuff to give 'em.' In spite of all I could say he got up and came down to the table. The lads, appalled at his ghastly appearance, tried to prevail on him to go back to bed, but he refused and when they persisted, he got cross and said he was alright. It was obvious he had a high fever, but he came out on the exercise ground and tried to play a game of rounders. He gritted his teeth and put the thing over him on his feet. In three days he was his old normal self.[72]

Padraic Colum's account of Griffith and the flu is remarkably similar to that of Brennan:

> One morning Denis McCullough encountered Arthur Griffith on the iron stairway. 'You've got influenza!' McCullough cried, startled by Griffith's appearance. 'I can handle it', he replied. 'How?' 'Quinine.' 'How much have you taken?' 'The whole bottle.' McCullough was alarmed for Griffith's eyes were protuberant and the veins on his head

were enlarged. He thought Griffith would collapse from the remedy as much as from the disease. Whatever state he was in it did not stop him playing handball and attending on other prisoners who could not get about.'[73]

At forty-eight years old, Griffith was one of the older internees. Yet he had a reputation for his physical strength and fitness, a result of his early gymnastic training, regular cycling and daily swim. Before contracting influenza, he was considered so fit that he had been chosen as the best physical candidate for a planned escape over a sixteen-foot wall, using rope made out of linen towels (linen fibres are particularly tough). Part of the plan involved scaling another ten-foot wall with no apparent foothold. Griffith's insistence on fighting the flu 'on his feet' may have contributed to the breakdown in his health that led to his premature death on 12 August 1922.[74] P.S. O'Hegarty described his premature death as something that had seemed unlikely during the jail years. 'Whoever else died, we felt sure it should not be Griffith – Griffith with the iron will, the iron constitution, the imperturbable nerve; Griffith whom we all thought certain to live to be one hundred and write the epitaphs of all.'[75] The influenza pandemic cast long shadows.

O'Hegarty makes the argument that the 'German' plot through the removal of the standing committee of Sinn Féin from circulation, made Collins a political force. He suggests that it was at this time that the movement as a whole became aware of him, sensed his personality and his leadership, began to admire him and to have the level of trust in him which hitherto they had placed in Griffith and de Valera. 'And so, when the prisoners came out after the failure of the plot, they found a new leader. They found Collins doing everything and leading everywhere, and trusted by everybody.'[76] The commonplace post-influenzal malaise and the frequent and sometimes severe sequelae of this influenza may have also affected the post-release performance of some internees. A Sinn Féin pamphlet published in 1919 claimed that many were broken in health, some so seriously that no hope was entertained of their complete recovery.[77]

The influenza epidemic is frequently discussed in the Bureau of Military History witness statements, a State-collected archive of recollections of activists during Ireland's revolutionary period. The nursing role played by Cumann na mBan during the period often appears magnified by historians compared to the evidence from the witness statements. Similarly, Kathleen Lynn's work, while of good intent, does not seem to be as influential or large in scale as the attention it receives would suggest. Lynn's diary shows she opened her influenza hospital in October, cleared out the last of the patients before Christmas on 18 December, and it remained closed for several months during the epidemic, until she reopened it on 9 March 1919, frustrated that she could do so little to help otherwise. Her typically terse diary notes for 6 March 1919 read: 'the flu rages, I can do little, poor children & all dying around. Miss Jellett better. Mrs Clarke fine'. Kathleen Clarke, whose health often gave cause for concern, caught influenza after her release from Holloway. The Charlemont facility seems to have been quite modest, from the comments in Lynn's diary.

Ian Miller observes that one of the Bureau's contributors, Sean Moylan, portrays his influenza experience and his soldiering in the revolution as facing 'two simultaneous battles: one physical, one military' and that in Moylan's view, both influenza and Britain are enemies that had to be conquered. In Miller's reading of Moylan's witness statement, Moylan, as a soldier, presents himself as having battled physical discomfort to pursue republican activity, subordinating his personal suffering from influenza to the national interest.[78]

Historians writing about Irish politics during this time have tended, until McConville and Murphy's important works on political imprisonment, to ignore or ascribe only a peripheral role to the influenza epidemic. Others seldom give the epidemic even a peripheral mention in connection with the 1918 general election, which was a game changer for Irish separatism. And yet, the elements of the political situation most influenced by the influenza epidemic – conscription, the 'German' plot, and the 1918 election – combined, as P.S. O'Hegarty wrote, to throw more and more elements in the country over to Sinn Féin. The weight of influence the Spanish flu had on the political situation and in particular on the pivotal December 1918 general election is open to conjecture. It does seem logical, from a study of the sources viewed here, that Sinn Féin, when presented with this *deus ex machina*, constructed a potent influenza narrative which highlighted the supposedly dire conditions under which the internees were being detained and the breakdown in health that many of them had endured. Sinn Féin made a conscious decision to harness the illness and deaths among Irish political prisoners from influenza to hammer home the message they wanted to convey to both the Irish people and the British administration. The influenza epidemic was a critical factor in reversing the Government's success in subverting the anti-conscription campaigners by removing them from circulation. Influenza helped to prove the theory promoted by Sinn Féin that the conditions under which the internees were being detained were hazardous to their health, even though statistics on death from influenza in prisons generally would suggest that the prisoners were actually safer than they would have been at large. William Murphy has described imprisonment as one of the fundamental ways in which nationalists identified themselves as rebels and shaped their resistance. 'Imprisonment provided them with an identity, with status, with an opportunity to rebel, with publicity. For them, their incarceration, suffering and struggle made flesh the bondage of their country, sex or class and became an instrument of revolution.'[79] The outbreaks of influenza among internees and political prisoners in British and Irish jails at the very least enhanced the opportunity to publicise that bondage and to play on public opinion at a crucial time in Irish political history.

Notes

1 William Murphy, *Political Imprisonment and the Irish* (Oxford: Oxford University Press, 2014), pp. 82–8.
2 Ben Novick, 'Propaganda I: Advanced nationalist propaganda and moralistic revolution, 1914–1918', in Joost Augusteijn, ed., *The Irish Revolution, 1913–1923* (Basingstoke: Palgrave, 2002), pp. 34–52. Virginia Glandon, *Arthur Griffith and the Advanced Nationalist Press: Ireland, 1900–1922* (New York: Peter Lang, 1985).
3 *Midland Tribune*, 26 October and 2 November 1918.
4 Fearghal McGarry, *The Rising – Ireland: Easter 1916* (Oxford: Oxford University Press, 2011), pp. 91–2.
5 Ibid., p. 276.
6 Thomas J. Brophy 'On Church Grounds: Political Funerals and the Contest to Lead Catholic Ireland', *The Catholic Historical Review*, vol. 95, no. 3 (July 2009), pp. 491–514.
7 GPB, 1918/7585; GPB, 1918/8243; GPB, 1918/7941.
8 *Belfast Prison inquiry. Report by the Right Honourable Mr. Justice Dodd of the proceedings at the inquiry directed by the Special Commission (Belfast Prison) Act, 1918* (1919), xxvii, cmd 83. DORA, or the Defence of the Realm Act, 1914, was introduced to curtail activity which was seen as a threat to sovereignty from the beginning of the world war.

9 GPB, 1919/268.

10 GPB, 1918/6687.

11 CSORP, 1918 28583.

12 CSORP, 1918 28634, 28544, 28426.

13 GPB, 1918/6739.

14 GPB, 1918/6970.

15 GPB, 1918/6895.

16 GPB, 1918/7449.

17 GPB, 1918/8075.

18 GPB, 1918/8277.

19 See *Irish Times* issues throughout January 1919 for details of roof protest by prisoners in Belfast jail, over restrictions on their conditions since the flu. GPB 1919/ 2215.

20 Alan J. Ward, 'America and the Irish Problem 1899–1921', *Irish Historical Studies*, xvi, no. 61 (March 1968), pp. 64–90.

21 Michael T. Foy, *Michael Collins's Intelligence War* (Stroud: Sutton, 2006).

22 Murphy, *Political Imprisonment and the Irish*, pp. 108–9.

23 William Murphy, 'The state, the law and political imprisonment, 1914–1918', www.rte.ie/centuryireland/index.php/articles/the-state-the-law-and-political-imprisonment-1914–1918 (accessed 21 January 2017).

24 Michael Laffan, *The Resurrection of Ireland* (Cambridge: Cambridge University Press, 1999), pp. 142–5. The arrests were permitted under the Defence of the Realm Act. Few authorities agree on the exact number arrested the first day or detained overall, as even as some were being picked up, others were being let go because of illness or family circumstances.

25 CO 904/164. Various letters to and from the interned prisoners mention this issue.

26 CO904/164.

27 Murphy, *Political Imprisonment and the Irish*, p. 264.

28 Sean McConville, *Irish Political Prisoners 1848–1922* (London: Routledge, 2003), p. 638.

29 CO 904, 186. A letter, undated but from December 1918, from TC Kingsmill Moore on behalf of the press censor to the editors of all Irish newspapers said that all communications from Irish internees in Great Britain should be submitted to the press censor's office before publication.

30 *Irish Independent*, 28 October 1918.

31 Royal College of Physicians in Ireland heritage centre: Kathleen Lynn diaries.

32 Margaret Ó hÓgartaigh, *Kathleen Lynn – Irishwoman, Patriot, Doctor* (Dublin: Irish Academic Press, 2006), passim. Bureau of Military History, Kathleen Lynn, Witness Statement 357.

33 CO904/164. Various letters to and from the interned prisoners mention this issue.

34 CO904/164. The internees' correspondence was read by the postal censor 4 March 1919, when the cabinet decided to release them.

35 CO 904/186.

36 Honor Ó Brolcháin and Geraldine Plunkett Dillon, *All in the Blood* (Dublin: A & A Farmar, 2006), pp. 265–6.

37 *Midland Tribune*, 19 October 1918.

38 CO 904/186.

39 Bureau of Military History, Maud Gonne, Witness Statement 317.

40 CO904/164.

41 Murphy, *Political Imprisonment and the Irish*, pp. 115–16. Murphy gives an excellent account of the internees' lives in prison.

42 CO904/164.

43 Bureau of Military History, Maud Gonne, Witness Statement 317.

44 *Irish Independent*, 24 January 1919.

45 Propaganda (Sinn Féin) pamphlets. National Library, accession no. IR 94109, Number 3, 'Two years of English atrocities in Ireland, 1917–1918.'

46 The postal censor said that correspondence after the death of Coleman showed that it was being exploited as 'a further instance of British inhumanity'. CO904/164. See also Frank Gallagher, *The Four Glorious Years 1918–1921* (Tallaght: Blackwater Press, 2005). *Irish Independent*, 12 December 1918.

47 CO 904/164.

48 CO 904/164.

49 CO 904/164.

50 M. Spillane from his mother, dated 13.12.18. CO 904/164.

51 Gallagher, *The Four Glorious Years 1918–1921*, pp. 51–4.

52 *Evening Herald*, 13 December 1918.

53 Frank Gallagher, *The Four Glorious Years 1918–1921* (Tallaght: Blackwater Press, 2005), p. 54. Áine Ceannt was the widow of 1916 rebellion leader Eamon Ceannt.

54 Royal College of Physicians in Ireland heritage centre: Kathleen Lynn diaries.

55 For the funeral report, see *Irish Independent*, 16 December 1918.

56 McConville, *Irish Political Prisoners 1848–1922*, pp. 650–1. Funeral report, *Irish Independent*, 12 December 1918.

57 CO 904/186.

58 Gallagher, *The Four Glorious Years 1918–1921*, p. 55.

59 P.S. O'Hegarty, *The Victory of Sinn Féin – How It Won It and How It Used It* (Dublin: University College Dublin Press, 1924), p. 21.

60 Robert Brennan, *Allegiance* (Dublin: Browne and Nolan, 1950), p. 167; Gallagher, *The Four Glorious Years 1918–1921*, p. 54.

61 Sinn Féin pamphlet collection, the National Library of Ireland: 'The case of Ireland' (1919).

62 *Weekly Irish Times*, 12 April 1919. Patrick Maume, 'French, Sir John', *Dictionary of Irish Biography*, http://dib.cambridge.org/viewReadPage. do?articleId=a3364; another irony: Edward Shortt's death in 1935 was from septicaemia following influenza.

63 *Irish Independent*, 3 March 1919.

64 Bureau of Military History, witness statement WS702: Frank Drohan, Clonmel, Co. Tipperary (p. 41).

65 *Irish Independent*, 3 March 1919.

66 Brennan, *Allegiance*, pp. 231–3.

67 *Irish Independent*, 7 March 1918.

68 Ó Brolcháin, *All in the Blood*. Deaglan Ó Bric, 'Pierce McCan MP. Part 1, 1882–1916' in *Tipperary Historical Journal*, 1988, pp. 121–32.

69 *Irish Independent*, 7 March 1919.

70 Thomas Ashe died on hunger strike in September 1917.

71 For more on Pierce McCan, see Deaglan Ó Bric, 'Pierce McCan, M.P. (1882–1919)', *The Tipperary Historical Journal*, 1989.

72 Brennan, *Allegiance*, pp. 233 and 229.

73 Colum, *Arthur Griffith*, p. 191.

74 Ibid., pp. 190–1.

75 P.S. O'Hegarty, *The Victory of Sinn Féin – How It Won It and How It Used It* (Dublin: UCD Press, 1998), p. 93.

76 Ibid., p. 19.

77 Sinn Féin Pamphlet collection, National Library of Ireland, 'The case of Ireland' (1919).

78 Ian Miller, 'Pain trauma and memory in the Irish War of Independence', in Fionnuala Dillane, Naomi McAreavey and Emilie Pine, eds, *The Body in Pain in Irish Literature and Culture* (Basingstoke: Palgrave MacMillan, 2016), pp. 117, 134.

79 William Murphy, 'The Tower of Hunger: political imprisonment and the Irish 1910–1921' (PhD thesis, UCD, 2006). See also Murphy, *Political Imprisonment and the Irish*, for an excellent account of internee life during the 'German' plot.

9

Epilogue: the long aftermath

'The past is never dead', William Faulkner wrote in *Requiem for a Nun*. 'It's not even past.'[1]

In the spring of 2009, as a PhD candidate researching Spanish influenza in an Irish context, I watched the unfolding of the Mexican influenza story with an almost obsessive interest. It was evident that fear had become a big part of that story, just as in 1918. When the news first broke, on 25 April 2009, an Air France captain refused to fly a plane from Paris to Mexico City. My then husband, a travel journalist heading to a Mexican travel trade fair in Acapulco, was on the plane. 'Check the news, it's like 1918!' he texted from the tarmac. In Benito Juárez airport, he texted again: 'You should come here to write, you'd get an idea of the panic.' Expatriate parents were rushing around, trying desperately to put their families onto flights out of the city to just about anywhere, and sometimes resorting in desperation to bribing the airline counter staff. As he had missed his connecting flights and all flights out of the airport were now full, he caught an atypically almost empty bus to Acapulco, as people stayed indoors, afraid of catching flu. The Mexican tourism industry – a key component in Mexico's economy earning $13.3 billion with 22 million visitors in 2008 – was effectively shut down, even though the main tourism centre of Cancún was at the far side of the country from Mexico City, where influenza was most concentrated. Access was curtailed as government advisories cautioned against or banned travel to Mexico. Airlines cancelled services. Travellers from Mexico were treated with extreme caution, and in some cases even sent back. Many of my husband's colleagues had to take circuitous routes home. The red-top newspapers and more responsible media alike rushed to find pictures of crowds wearing masks, and to devise scare-mongering headlines. The Mexican newspaper *Milenio's* front-page headline on 28 April 2009 read 'Ya es nivel 4! Inutil cerar fronteras' ('It's already level 4! Useless to close borders', which was a reference to the WHO pandemic scale). I confess to adding to the red-tops' scare-mongering flu stories in a 2,000-word article about the relevance of the 1918 pandemic to the contemporary crisis for the *Irish Daily Mail*. It is not often that a PhD student is asked to write for a tabloid newspaper, but high-profile television documentaries about the 1918–19 pandemic on history channels had primed the public to believe that another major influenza pandemic was overdue.

The panic surrounding the Mexican outbreak was eerily similar to what I was uncovering about the other 'Hispanic' influenza. In June 1918 – within days of the reporting of an unusually severe outbreak of influenza in Spain – the flu had arrived in Ireland, affecting mainly eastern Ulster and Dublin. Children were sent from Dublin and other cities to their relations in the country, which would give them a better chance of evading the disease. Adults huddled together, talking about this terrible thing that was about to befall them. People carried handkerchiefs and scarves dowsed in eucalyptus oil to act as a prophylactic when they went out in public. Editorials in newspapers were filled with dire warnings about this 'mystery malady' that had landed apparently from Spain, although there were whisperings of it coming also from other places, and a shocking rumour that even the Allied army had contracted it. The continual danger of reinfection during the epidemic period reinforced the level of fear clinging to the disease. Tommy Christian, when asked why the influenza was not spoken about in the long aftermath, said: 'Why would we speak about it? It kept coming back again, and again and again, so when it was not there we did not talk about it for fear it might come back again.' He has probably pinpointed a key reason for the initial reluctance to record the disease in history. Nobody wanted, in the immediate aftermath, to assess the damage. Contemporary medicine had failed to protect people from this disease, which had, as Michael Worboys observes, challenged the 'sense that contagious and infectious diseases were being tamed', at last.[2] Confidence in the new medical bacteriology had been severely dented.

Some of the puzzling reported features of this 2009 strain – the vulnerability of young adults and the rapid transmission – were evocative of the 1918–19 crisis. Fearful (and perhaps experiencing a little anticipatory excitement) that the world was about to experience another disease event on the scale of that awesome pandemic, 'experts' were produced by broadcast media and the popular press to discuss the likelihood of a pandemic reoccurring on the scale of that of 1918–19, and about other perceived facts gleaned from those hyperbolic documentaries on Spanish influenza. For example, some of them seized on the concept that pandemics always occur in waves, even though there was little evidence of wave patterns in the other two twentieth-century influenza pandemics, the Asian flu of 1957–58 or the Hong Kong pandemic of 1968–69. The talk that the 2009 pandemic would reoccur in waves inspired David Morens and Jeffrey Taubenberger to publish a study of the three twentieth-century pandemics and another eleven influenza pandemics since 1510, showing that there was little evidence in any other pandemic of a wave pattern similar to that of the 1918–19 epidemic, with numerous waves in less than a year (as distinguished from the expected annual recurrences typical of early post-pandemic and seasonal influenza).[3] The 1889–90 pandemic recurred annually for up to four years, but the recurrence intervals were all about one year or more apart; in the Northern Hemisphere they usually occurred between October and April (in the usual seasonal influenza period). Morens and Taubenberger concluded, from the findings of that study, that it was impossible to predict the trajectory of a pandemic of influenza based on the evidence from previous pandemics. The study proved, as they argued, that each event of pandemic influenza had to be lived forward but was best understood backwards.

Interpreting new epidemics of disease

Perhaps it might be helpful here to show how historians of disease can see broad but remarkably consistent patterns in how societies develop an understanding of emerging large-scale epidemics of infectious disease. Charles Rosenberg and other historians of medicine and disease have proposed that a major epidemic disease could be viewed as a dramaturgic event.[4] Rosenberg developed this interpretative framework for understanding a dramaturgy of disease: in Act I there came the progressive revelation, with communities slow to acknowledge its presence. Only when the acknowledgement of

disease became unavoidable was there public admission of its exist-
ence, with the public, physicians and authorities all reluctant to admit
the presence of such a potentially dangerous intruder. Act II saw the
creation of a framework within which its dismaying arbitrariness can
be managed; he called it 'Managing randomness'. Act III presented the
public response. For Rosenberg, one of the defining characteristics
of an epidemic was the pressure it generated for decisive and visible community response. Response did not necessarily mean taking
action to deal with the crisis, it could also mean doing nothing. He
said that the adoption and administration of public health measures
inevitably reflected cultural attitudes. In Act IV, epidemics normally end by fizzling out almost without notice. The disease became
endemic; the people had some degree of immunity. Yet the end of the
disease provided an implicit moral structure that could be imposed
as an epilogue. The epilogue, in Rosenberg's drama, assessed the
response of the community and its components to the challenge of
the epidemic. Historians and others, he observed, tended to look
back and ask what 'lasting impacts' epidemic disease events made
and what 'lessons' had been learned. Did the dead die in vain? Had
a heedless society reverted to its accustomed ways of doing things
as soon as the event passed? Rosenberg said that often there was an
implicit moral agenda to the scholarly interpretation of an epidemic,
and that epidemics have always implied an opportunity for retro-
spective moral judgement.[5] We can see this even today, as epidemics
of cholera in Haiti and of Ebola and other diseases in Africa are
considered indicative of the first world's failure to share its expertise
and wealth with poorer societies, while in the past colonial interpret-
ations of disease in Africa tended to blame the 'ignorance' of indi-
genous populations.

Major epidemic disease events test, support, undermine or reshape
social, political and medical assumptions and attitudes, and as Paul
Slack has explained, the study of past epidemics therefore throws 'a
peculiarly sharp light' on the ideologies and mentalities of the societies they afflicted.[6] Large epidemics challenge systems within society
and sometimes provide the impetus to change systems which have
needed change for years. Improvements to Irish and international
public health in the nineteenth century were generally reactive to disease incidents rather than to concepts emerging from developments
in medical science.

Niall Johnson has noted that in the aftermath of the pandemic, New Zealand and South Africa instigated commissions inquiring into the influenza and the responses to it; similarly, he observed, the development of public health systems in France, Australia, India, Iran and Russia could also be viewed as a consequence of the epidemic. In Canada, the influenza provided the impetus to establish a long awaited central health bureau, associated with a national laboratory.[7] In England and Wales, the LGB kept quite a low profile during the epidemic according to Johnson, issuing the occasional memorandum with advice on how to treat and to avoid influenza, and generally leaving their medical officers of health and local authorities to take whatever action they thought appropriate. One of the few actions they took was the eventual release of some doctors from military service to help the civilian population fight the flu. Seen in this context, the Irish Local Government Board's inactivity during the pandemic highlighted in earlier chapters was in keeping with the actions or lack of actions of their England and Wales counterpart. Johnson observed that even though some used the passivity of the LGB for England and Wales during the pandemic to enhance their calls for a new Ministry of Health, the ministry was not a new idea forged out of the influenza crisis but part of a pre-existing movement towards health reform.[8] It would seem, however, that George Newman, who had been appointed to the position of chief medical officer of the new Ministry of Health in England in 1919 as well as being principal medical officer of the Local Government Board for England and Wales, had insisted that the new Ministry should appoint more medical staff to deal with certain prevalent diseases, including influenza and tuberculosis, and that the 'many new rearrangements', which he had found from experience to be necessary to handle these diseases properly, were made.[9]

The death toll in from the 1918–19 influenza pandemic in Ireland (which spanned eleven months), at a conservative estimate of 20,000, exceeded the death toll of 19,000 from cholera in 1832, the year with the highest mortality rate in the 1832–35 cholera epidemic, a subject which has received a lot more attention of historians. By using the known death toll and a death rate of 2.5 per cent for those who caught the disease to calculate the morbidity or level of illness from the disease, I have estimated the likely morbidity or numbers of ill, suggesting that about one fifth of Ireland's population suffered from the disease, or 800,000 people, placing the Irish experience of Spanish influenza on a par with conservative estimates of the international morbidity from the disease. This work has shown that the populations of five Leinster counties, Kildare, Dublin, Wicklow, Wexford and Carlow, and of five Ulster counties, Antrim, Down, Armagh, Monaghan and Donegal, suffered the highest death tolls from influenza in the country in 1918 and 1919. It has also shown, that although more people died from this influenza in Ulster than in Leinster, Leinster had a slightly higher death rate per thousand of living population. In addition, this work has shown that children under the age of five and adults aged between twenty-five and thirty-five were more likely to die from the disease than any other age groups. Using weekly death statistics for Dublin in 1918–19 to identify the waves of the influenza epidemic, it has found that people who belonged to what the RG called the general service class suffered the highest death rates per thousand of living population. It has also shown that Dublin residents who worked in jobs where they came into close contact with others were more likely to die than those who did not; doctors and nurses, prison warders, police, postal workers, priests, hawkers, porters and their families were particularly at risk. By investigating rising death rates from other respiratory diseases during one of the peak weeks of the influenza epidemic, it has proved that there is reasonable evidence to suggest that the RG's final tally for deaths from the influenza may be an underestimate, particularly in relation to children under the age of five.

The disease challenged and dented the competence and confidence of the medical profession, whose scientific knowledge, skills and medicines proved less than up to the task of healing their patients when faced with such a difficult and protean disease. The chapter on the medical profession and the influenza epidemic has shown that doctors debated and disagreed on the nature of the disease, and on the methods and drugs required to treat it. Some became fascinated by the challenges it posed, and like William Boxwell, worked tirelessly to investigate it or to cure patients. In its aftermath, it was widely recognised, as the interviews with survivors in Chapter 7 and other material in this work have told, that good nursing was the best treatment, with plenty of liquids and when the patient had sufficiently recovered, nourishing food. In those areas where the influenza presented a major threat to the community, schemes were formed on an ad hoc basis by community organisations, local authorities, landlords and kind and brave neighbours to nurse the ill and to feed them and their families. These local responses were recognised to have been instrumental in saving many lives.

Within the independence movement, influenza was adopted as a political tool by Sinn Féin propagandists, and may have enhanced its success in the 1918 general election. The organisation used its contacts within the national and regional press to persuade the people that the detention of many of the Sinn Féin leadership and prominent anti-conscription campaigners in jails in England and Wales was both unjust and potentially harmful to their health, because of the prison conditions. When Richard Coleman of Swords in north Co. Dublin died in the days immediately preceding the general election, Sinn Féin election workers moved swiftly to incorporate his death into their election material, adding his name to the list of Sinn Féin 'martyrs' and decorating the election posters and banners with black ribbons in his honour. The organisation claimed his death in jail from influenza as yet another act in the list of perceived injustices by the British Government towards the Irish people. It also took advantage of the propagandist opportunity provided by deaths of their supporters from influenza or influenzal pneumonia to write hagiographical obituaries in the regional press. Whether Sinn Féin's eager adoption of the influenza epidemic as a propaganda tool had a major effect in persuading the electorate to support their candidates is impossible to gauge, but its influence is worth considering. Because of its timing, in the wake of the establishment of the First Dáil, Pierce McCan's death had a different kind of influence. It offered nationalists the opportunity to participate in large numbers in the pageantry at which they excelled. It permitted a passive show of people power and confidence, an indication of change. The disease seemed to provide well-timed opportunities to tip the balance of public opinion in favour of the radical nationalist movement and away from the Irish Parliamentary Party, the LGB and the Government.

This study has also argued that the influenza epidemic, by placing pressure on the medical system and its institutions, threw its own 'peculiarly sharp light' on pre-existing tensions between the LGB and the BOGs as local administrators of the Poor Law medical system, and highlighted problems over the terms and conditions of the employment of the Poor Law medical officers of health. These included the shortage of doctors available to work for the Poor Law medical system, because of the embargo on employing doctors young enough to work for the armed forces. The epidemic further-more highlighted poor levels of communication and understanding between the LGB and their various agents. According to Mary Daly, the LGB regarded the minutes of the Poor Law BOGs as the 'prin-cipal medium of correspondence between the boards of guardians and the Commissioners', enabling the latter to at once interpose their authority when any irregular or unauthorised proceedings took place or were contemplated.[10] This communications system clearly did not work all that successfully during the influenza epidemic, and the problem may have been compounded by the deteriorating rela-tionship between the BOGs, which were increasingly nationalist in composition, and an LGB that was seen as being increasingly out of touch with the needs of the people. It has revealed, through the extra pressure placed on hospital beds, that most hospitals were facing acute financial difficulties caused by inadequate funding, by the pressure of accommodating sick soldiers and by substantial increases in the price of many commodities – including medicine, coal, bread, grain, pota-toes, sugar and alcohol.

Spanish influenza was the last great crisis to face the LGB and a disjointed medical system which had received harsh criticism over the previous fifty years. The claimed responses of the LGB were limited; even their decision to provide a free vaccine was lethargic and ineffective, coming as it did at the end of the epidemic: the Indian Government had been providing a free vaccine since December 1918, basing its formulation on research information provided by the War Office.[11] The influenza epidemic highlighted various problems within the health system, many of which had been discussed in earlier reappraisals of various aspects of the system. The influenza could be considered to be part of a process in which the authority of the LGB, the most powerful organ of the British administration in Ireland, was undermined.[12] Laurence Geary has observed that despite some moves to change the health system by the Vice-Regal Commission on Poor Law Reform in 1906 and the Royal Commission on the Poor Laws in 1909, and also the widespread dissatisfaction with the system voiced through the pages of the medical journals, the unreformed health system 'limped along for another ten years until 1920, when the Irish Health Council called for reform'.[13] The reforms proposed by the commissions were shelved when the First World War broke out.[14] The topic of Irish health reform was a source of constant discussion in the *Medical Press* and the *British Medical Journal*. Thomas Hennessy's article on medical reform for Ireland considered how the Irish medical situation could be fitted into a new Ministry of Health, similar to that proposed for England and Wales. His main proposal was that all functions relating to health would be centralised into one department, unlike the disjointed system that existed in 1919, and this move should be accompanied by a total reform of the Poor Law medical system.[15]

The Irish epilogue to Spanish influenza?

No direct mention was made of the influenza epidemic, Ireland's most recent acute health crisis, and the most traumatic since the cholera epidemic associated with the Great Famine, in the report of the Irish Public Health Council (1920).[16] And yet, from a close reading of the report, it would appear that the influenza crisis, having cast that 'peculiarly sharp light' on malfunctions within the healthcare system, did indeed inform many of the recommendations. The council was constituted in the immediate aftermath of the influenza – its first meeting was in October 1919 – to advise the chief secretary about a comprehensive reform of the health services in preparation for submitting a bill to Parliament. The pandemic crisis, and the failings of the healthcare system that it highlighted, were still fresh memories. Initially, there were fears that its membership would not reflect a broad spectrum of interested parties, including those critical of the Government's handling of Irish health crises, but these fears proved unfounded. There were seven medical members of the seventeen-member board, which was chaired by Dr Edward Coey Bigger, medical commissioner of the LGB. The other medical members were Dr E.F. Stephenson, acting medical commissioner of the LGB, Dr W.J. Maguire, medical commissioner of the Insurance Commission, RG Sir William Thompson, Sir William Moore of the Royal Academy of Medicine in Ireland, and Dr R.J. Rowlette and Dr Alice Barry as direct representatives of the council of the Irish medical profession. Other members included Sir Henry Robinson, the vice-president of the LGB, the chairman and a commissioner of the Irish Insurance Commission, representatives of approved societies, insurance and tuberculosis committees, veterinary medical associations and nursing institutions. The council considered the recommendations made by the Vice-Regal Commission, the Royal Commission, and by the departmental committee that was appointed in 1913 to look at extending medical insurance benefits to Ireland, as well as recommendations from the medical profession and health insurance societies. Its astute findings and recommendations for a comprehensive overhaul of the country's medical systems met with the approval of the medical profession, including Hennessy.[17]

The report noted that there was a 'considerable lack of co-ordination, and a certain amount of overlapping, both in the central control and local administration of the public health services', and that several departments within the Irish Government structures were dealing 'more or less independently' with issues to do with health. It observed that few people, apart from the officials directly involved, understood the 'enormously complicated system of local health administration'. The report was quite blunt in its reflections on the shambolic nature of the top-level administration of the existing systems, describing it as 'uneconomical and unsound', because of the lack of co-ordination and overlapping of duties between the various structures. The council recommended that there should be complete co-ordination in the central administration of the mental and public health services in Ireland. In a clause that seems to be directly aimed at the LGB's constitutional failure to communicate with other stakeholders, highlighted during the influenza crisis, the council observed that it was essential to the successful administration of any central health authority that it should be in close communication with the public authorities, medical profession and the various semi-official and voluntary organisations that are interested in the health conditions of the people. The report added a telling rider that the council considered it an urgent matter to establish a central health authority that was 'in close touch with public opinion and with the various interests concerned'. This echoed the constant criticisms of the LGB for its failure to communicate or to understand that the pandemic required a different sort of management, as noted in several instances earlier in this book.

All the various medical services should, the report suggested, be co-ordinated centrally on a county basis. It further recommended that the dispensary medical system should be completely removed from the Poor Law administration, and remodelled with the area of local control extended from the union to the county, and unified with the proposed general county medical and hospital system. It proposed that the new system would then cater to both the poor and insured workers. The committee advocated the unification of the disjointed hospital system, under the county health authority, and simplifying the very complicated admission systems. It noted the financial difficulties that the voluntary hospitals were experiencing, and suggested that these hospitals should be given some financial assistance to enable them to continue functioning.[18] In what was probably an oblique reference to the influenza crisis, it recommended that the Acts relating to the notification of infectious disease – the Infectious Disease Act (1889), the Infectious Disease (Prevention) Act (1890), and Part IV of the Public Health Acts Amendments Act (1907) – be made mandatory rather than allowing their permissive character to continue. It criticised the lack of research facilities in Ireland, which was a point that had also been made by the LGB in its annual reports in relation to the epidemic. It strongly advised that funds be provided to carry out a comprehensive system of medical research under the direction of an Irish Ministry of Health, and further recommended that medical officers be required to record the results of their practice to pass on their knowledge to scientific investigators. Its suggestions relating to the doctors employed within the reformed dispensary system also resonate with the issues about doctors' pay and pensions raised during the influenza crisis. It proposed the establishment of an Irish medical service with opportunities for promotion, entitlements to superannuation and a formal pay structure, rather than the ad hoc system administered by the BOGs.

But yet again, the much-needed changes to the medical systems were deferred, as the change in governance intervened. In 1920, Dáil Éireann set up a new local government department, which co-existed with the LGB until 1922, with an increasing number of BOGs opting to align with the Dáil's department. The process of changing the system was delayed yet again, although many of the recommendations of the Irish Public Health Council were eventually adopted over a period of years.[19] Ruth Barrington has stressed that while the years preceding independence were dominated by the struggle for independence, and that while histories of the period usually concentrate on political and military events, it would be misleading to suggest that every facet of Irish life was equally affected by those events and that nothing much else of consequence happened during the period. The years from 1913 onwards were, she advocated, 'seminal for the future direction and administration of the health services.' She urged that the sense of continuity between the periods before and after independence for the development of the Irish health services ought not to be overemphasised.[20] Whether or not the influenza epidemic really influenced the changes that were eventually made is open to conjecture, but it would seem that influenza, as Paul Slack theorised in relation to major epidemics of disease in general, cast a 'peculiar light' on the malfunctions within the Irish medical 'system' and thus made it easier to see the changes that were necessary.

'Spanish' influenza as a model for future pandemics

The Spanish influenza pandemic continues to have a contemporary impact on public health policy, as international and national bodies use data from it to project figures for a worst-case scenario in the event of future influenza pandemics. Towards the end of the twentieth century, medical experts speculated that the development of a new influenza virus with pandemic potential was imminent, with their fears stimulated by the outbreaks of SARS and the highly morbid Influenza A H5N1 or avian influenza. Health agencies prepared national and international strategies to manage a new pandemic of influenza, using projection models to suggest likely outcomes for future pandemics. In Ireland, the Pandemic Influenza Expert Group chaired by Professor William Hall, director of the National Virus Reference Laboratory, published a report 'Modelling impact of pandemic influenza: interim report on use of empirical model in Ireland' in December 2006. The model was based on data from influenza deaths in England and Wales during the 1969–70 and 1957 pandemics and London during the 1918 pandemic.[21] In deriving predictions from the model they offered two different scenarios: the first with a clinical attack rate of 25 per cent and a mortality rate of 0.55 per cent; and the second with a clinical attack rate of 50 per cent and a mortality rate (in this case mortality rate means the death rate among clinical cases of influenza, which is sometimes referred to as the case fatality rate) of 2.5 per cent. The first scenario predicted that there would be 3,217 deaths, taking the Republic's population as 4.23 million, while the second scenario predicted 52,937 deaths; both predictions were based on a fifteen-week interval. This study used figures from London to devise a model for an influenza pandemic in an Irish scenario. Wartime London, with its possible proximity to the site of origin of the 1918 pandemic, large numbers of soldiers passing through on their way to and from the arena of war, and its densely housed population, whose health was undermined by war-time deprivation and stress, had a peculiar set of conditions which would not have applied in late twentieth-century Ireland or Dublin. The weekly influenza death statistics available for Dublin during the 1918–19 pandemic, which are used in Chapter 3, might have been a more logical and authentic choice for the model.[22]

One cannot help feeling that the major impact of the influenza pandemic was not on politics, medicine, government structures, or public health administration, but on private lives. Individuals and families suffered from loss, altered economic circumstances and changed family structures, and even for those on whom it did not directly impact, fear in the face of an awesome and unconquerable enemy. The interviews gathered for this work make a contribution towards documenting that fear and the terrible tragedies, the sense of loss, the unfathomable sadness that remained with those who lost family members to it for the rest of their lives. The trauma of lost lives and altered family circumstances continued to trouble the people interviewed for this work throughout their lives. For many, recalling tragic deaths proved emotionally difficult even though the event had occurred ninety years earlier. Many also expressed a sense of relief at finding out at last, in the context of the interview, what it was all about. They had been through a terrifying experience, had suffered from illness, loss, or the threats of these, and had no way of evaluating what had happened in its larger contexts. Several asked eagerly for further information on the pandemic, as if by knowing the enemy, they could assess the war they had been through, rather than just the skirmish or even the battle. For Tommy Christian and others, knowing what took place in the national context helped to make sense of the trauma of what happened to his own family. The absence of a national influenza narrative of any sort, written or oral, elongated their trauma.

Memories of the traumatic effect that influenza had on family health informed and guided domestic medicine and nursing in the ensuing years. For years afterwards, the individual health of some sufferers was affected; as R.B. McDowell's interview documented, some people had to consider their career options while taking into account the damage caused to their bodies by the disease. R.B. himself was left with a life-long fascination with his own health that may well have been triggered by his early close call with death; and yet although he had been considered an invalid for most of his youth and early adulthood, he lived to extreme old age. Some interviewees recalled that in later years' precautions were still being taken that were reminiscent of the time when the threat of the pandemic was present; for example, when a seasonal influenza seemed to be getting particularly troublesome, local authorities would disinfect buses. Others pondered whether their parents' almost paranoid fears that they would 'catch' cold were a manifestation of post-pandemic trauma. Children were urged to wrap up well in layers of warm woolly clothing, and advised not to go out with their hair wet in case they 'caught a chill', evidence that while the medical profession might have claimed for the most part to have abandoned their belief in the theory of miasma, it had and continues to have deep roots in the beliefs of the populace. Unsubstantiated tales of mass burials during the influenza epidemic, particularly of children, abound.[23] Unlike some other countries with more detailed health and death statistics, the true extent of family loss in Ireland as a result of the pandemic will never be known, but it appears to be greater than the official statistics indicated.

The 1918–19 pandemic has legacies that still endure. It persuaded international health authorities of the need to set up the global influenza-monitoring system that exists today, which is run by the World Health Organization. It has left a physical imprint through the graves of the dead, the pages of cemetery records, and the thousands of news pages and new histories documenting its effects. Although most of the survivors have now died, it lingers in the memories of families whose lives it radically altered, when it killed or incapacitated their members, left families without a breadwinner, children orphaned and parents mourning the loss of their little ones.

Notes

1 William Faulkner, *Requiem for a Nun*. London: Chatto and Windus, 1919, p. 85.
2 Michael Worboys, 'Contagion', in Mark Jackson, ed., *The Routledge History of Disease* (Abingdon: Routledge, 2017), pp. 71–88.
3 David Morens and Jeffery Taubenberger, 'Understanding Influenza Backward', *Journal of the American Medical Association*, cccii, no. 6 (2009), pp. 679–80.
4 Finding common ground between many papers presented at the Past and Present conference on 'Epidemics and Ideas' held in Exeter College, Oxford, in September 1989, Richard Evans suggested that there might be a common 'dramaturgy' to all epidemic diseases. Terence Ranger and Paul Slack, eds, *Epidemics and Ideas; Essays On the Historical Perception of Pestilence* (Cambridge: Cambridge University Press, 1999), p. 3.
5 Charles Rosenberg,'Aids in historical perspective', in *Explaining Epidemics and Other Studies in the History of Medicine* (Cambridge: Cambridge University Press, 1992), pp. 280–7.
6 Paul Slack in Ranger and Slack, eds, *Epidemics and Ideas*, p. 3.
7 Niall Johnson, *Britain and the 1918–19 Influenza Pandemic – a Dark Epilogue* (Abingdon: Routledge), pp. 196–7.
8 Niall Johnson, 'Influenza in Britain in 1918–19', in Howard Phillips and David Killingray, eds, *The Spanish Influenza Pandemic of 1918–1919*, pp. 150–1.
9 Forty-eighth annual report of the Local Government Board (for England and Wales), 1918–1919, supplement containing the report of the Medical Department for 1918–19 (1919), cmd 462.
10 M. E. Daly, *The Buffer State – The Historical Roots of the Department of the Environment* (Dublin: Institute of Public Administration, 1997), p. 14.
11 Radula Ramona, 'The Bombay experience', in Phillips, Howard and Killingray, David, eds, *The Spanish Influenza Pandemic of 1918–1919*, pp. 86–98.
12 See Ruth Barrington, *Health, Medicine and Politics in Ireland 1900–1970* (Dublin: Institute of Public Administration, 2000), pp. 94–5.
13 Laurence Geary, 'Medicine and the State: The Poor Law medical service in Ireland, 1851–1921', in the Mackey Lecture series, National Library of Ireland, 9 February 2010.
14 Desmond Roche, *Local Government*, second edn (Dublin: Institute of Public Administration, 1963), p. 26.
15 Thomas Hennessy, 'Medical reform for Ireland', *British Medical Journal*, i, no. 3039 (29 March 1919).
16 *Report of the Irish Public Health Council on the Public Health and Medical Services in Ireland* (Parl. Papers 1920 (Cmd. 761), xvii).

17 See, e.g., Thomas Hennessy, 'The report of the Irish Public Health
    Council', *British Medical Journal*, i, no 3104 (26 June 1920), pp. 870–2.
18 See Chapter 4.
19 Roche, *Local Government*, pp. 28–9.
20 Barrington, *Health, Medicine and Politics in Ireland*, pp. 87–8.
21 Pandemic Influenza Expert Group, 'Modelling impact of pandemic influ-
    enza: interim report on use of empirical model in Ireland'. See www.ndsc.
    ie/hpsc/A-Z/EmergencyPlanning/AvianPandemicInfluenzaPreparedne
    ssforIreland/Suplement3toChapter3/File220.en.pdf December 2006.
22 Hall, William, 'Report on pandemic preparedness, 2007', in www.ucd.ie/
    news/jan07/011907_pandemic_report.htm, accessed 23 March 2007.
23 See, e.g., John Colgan and David Cormack, 'Leixlip-Confey Gravestones',
    in *Journal of the County Kildare Archaeological Society*, xix (Part III)
    (2004–5), p. 502.

Select bibliography

Primary sources

Archival sources

Colonial Office
Prison correspondence CO904/164.

National Archives of Ireland
Chief Secretary's Office Registered Papers (CSORP) 1918–19.
General Prisons Board Correspondence (GPB) 1918–19.
Dublin Union Board of Guardians minute books (BG), 1918–19.
Business records series 19/2/8, J. and E. Nichols' daybook for 1916–19.

National Archives, Kew
National Archives: WO35/1794. Call for historical review of medical work in the Irish command during the war period.

National Library of Ireland
Frank Gallagher papers.
Pierce McCan papers.
Propaganda (Sinn Féin) pamphlets:
'Two years of English atrocities in Ireland, 1917–1918.'
'The Case of Ireland' (1919).
Lynn, Kathleen, 'Report on influenza pandemic' to Ard-Fheis (extraordinary) Sinn Féin (1919).

Dublin City Archive
Dublin Corporation minute books.

Dublin Corporation reports and printed documents, "Report of the Public Health Committee re hospital accommodation for influenza-pneumonia cases', i (1919), p. 587.

Bureau of Military History

Witness statement WS702: Frank Drohan.
Witness statement WS317: Maud Gonne.
Glasnevin cemetery: burial ledgers.

Royal College of Physicians in Ireland Heritage Centre

Kathleen Lynn diaries.
Sir Patrick Dun's Hospital archive: post-mortem book.
The House of Recovery and Fever Hospital, Cork St, Dublin archive: medical report for the year ending 31 March 1920.

Russell Library, Maynooth University

Annual report of the President of St Patrick's College, Maynooth, 1918–19.

Trinity College Dublin

Manuscripts department, Adelaide Hospital Archive:
Sixty-first annual report of the Adelaide and Fetherston-Haugh convalescent home, Rathfarnham, for 1918.
Adelaide Hospital finance and house committee minutes, 1918.
Medical reports of the Adelaide Hospital for 1918 and 1919.

Clongowes Wood College

The minister's journal.
Pupil lists for 1918–19.
Clongownian, 1919 and 1920.

Allen Library

Kathleen Lynn papers.

Archive of the Catholic Archdiocese of Dublin

Correspondence of William Walsh, Archbishop of Dublin.

Irish Railway Records Society

Great Southern and Western Railway secretary's office files, annual report of the transport manager for 1918, GSWR Files 3027–3078, Irish Railway Records Society, Heuston Station, Dublin.

Kildare County Council Archive

Athy Board of Guardians Minute Books, 1918 and 1919.
Naas Board of Guardians Minute Books, 1918 and 1919.

Diaries

Lord Cloncurry (in private local hands), 1918.

Interviews and personal communications

Andrews, Rosalind, Dublin, 9 July 2007.
Boylan, Catherine, Celbridge, Co. Kildare, 20 November 2008.
Byrne, Hugh, Dublin and Mayo, series of telephone calls 2008–17.
Burke, Ann, Celbridge, Co. Kildare, series of telephone and email correspondence, 2007–17.
Christian, Tommy, Ardclough, Co. Kildare, 12 April 2007.
Claffey, Seamus, undertaker, Ferbane, Co. Offaly, November 2007.
Davitt, Eileen 'Bab', Ferns, Co. Wexford, February and July, 2008.
Deacon, Margaret, Enniscorthy, Co. Wexford, July 2007.
Doyle, Catherine, Lucan, Co. Dublin, February 2007.
Enid (full name and address with author), Dublin, July 2007.
Fitzgerald, John, Co. Meath, telephone communication, March 2008.
Gogarty, Joan, Naas, Co. Kildare, personal communication, October 2008.
Heatley, Fred, Dublin, series of telephone and email correspondence, 2008–17.
Higgins, Lena, Naas, Co. Kildare, July 2007.
Kelly, James, Belfast, 20 May 2010.
Molloy, Elizabeth, Lucan, Co. Dublin, January 2007.
McConnon Larkin, Stella, series of interviews and telephone calls, 2010–17.
McDowell, R.B., Trinity College, Dublin, December 2006.
McMenamin, Kathleen, October 2010, response to questionnaire by post, undated.
McNally Sheil, Mary, Rathcoole, Co. Dublin, April 2007.
O'Toole, Nellie, Merrion Road, Ballsbridge, Dublin, September 2008.
Ralph, Cissie, Ferns, Co. Wexford, August 2009.
Rynhart, Olive, Ferns. February 2007.
Shankey, Anne, Dublin, telephone call, March 2008.
Tubridy, Jim, Cooraclare, Co. Clare, November 2008.
Walsh, Dr James, Terenure, Dublin, December 2009.

At Brabazon Home, Dublin

January 2007:
Heuston, Elizabeth.
Salmon, Thomas NDC.

Taylor, Florrie.
Vaughan, Olive.

At Dominican Nursing Home, Cabra Road, Dublin
March 2007:
Callanan, Sr Wilfrid.
Sr Theresa.

At Larchfield nursing home, Naas, Co. Kildare
July 2007:
Higgins, Lena.

At The Moyne Nursing Home, Enniscorthy, Co. Wexford
July 2007:
Rowesome, Mary Anne.

Telephone calls in connection with Irish Times article
Sieve, Raphael.
Brady, Colm.
Shankey, Anne.
O'Sullivan, Noreen.
Macnamara, Maccon.
Fitzgerald, John.

Parliamentary papers and official reports

Weekly returns of births and deaths for the Dublin registration area and in eighteen of the principal urban districts by the registrar general for Ireland, 1918–20.

Quarterly summary of the weekly returns of births and deaths for the Dublin registration area and in eighteen of the principal urban districts by the registrar general, 1918–20.

Quarterly returns of births, deaths and marriages in provinces, counties, poor law unions, and registrars' districts in Ireland, 1918–20.

Fifty-fifth annual report of registrar-general for Ireland for 1918 (Births, Deaths, and Marriages) (1919), x, cmd 450.

Fifty-sixth annual report of registrar-general for Ireland for 1919 (Births, Deaths, and Marriages) (1920), xi, cmd 997.

Fifty-seventh annual report of registrar-general for Ireland for 1920 (Births, Deaths, and Marriages) (1921), cmd 1532.

Report of the National Health Insurance Commission (Ireland) on the administration of National Health Insurance in Ireland during the period November 1917, to 31 March 1920 (1921), xv, cmd 653.

Report of the National Health Insurance Commission (Ireland) on the administration of national health insurance in Ireland during the period November 1917, to 31 March, 1920 (1921), xv, cmd 1147.

Ministry of Health Act, 1919. Report of the Irish Public Health Council on the public health and medical services in Ireland (1920), xvii, cmd 761.

Sixty-eighth annual report of the Inspectors of Lunatics, for the year ending 31 December 1918 (1920), xxi, cmd 579.

Sixty-ninth annual report of the Inspectors of Lunatics (Ireland) for the year ending 31 December 1919 (1921), xv, cmd 1127.

Forty-seventh annual report of the Local Government Board for Ireland for the year ended 31 March 1919 (1920), xxi, cmd 578.

Forty-eighth annual report of the Local Government Board for Ireland, for the year ended 31 March 1920 (1921), xiv, cmd 1432.

Forty-eighth annual report of the Local Government Board [for England and Wales], *1918–1919* (1920), xxiv, cmd 413.

Supplement to the forty-eighth Local Government Board [for England and Wales] *annual report, containing the report of the medical department for 1918–1919* (1920), xxiv, cmd 462.

Influenza, a supplement to the eighty-first report of the registrar-general, on the mortality from influenza in England and Wales 1918–1919 (1920), x, cmd 700.

Forty-first report of the General Prisons Board, Ireland, 1918–1919 (1920), xxiii, cmd 687.

Forty-second report of the General Prisons Board, Ireland, 1919–1920 (1921), xvi, cmd 1375.

Belfast Prison inquiry: report by the Right Honorable Mr. Justice Dodd of the proceedings at the inquiry directed by the Special Commission (Belfast Prison) Act, 1918 (1919), xxvii, cmd 83.

Report of the prison commissioners for Scotland, for the year 1918 (1919), xxvii, cmd 78.

Report of the prison commissioners for Scotland, for the year 1919 (1920), xxiii, cmd 698.

Report of the commissioners of prisons and the directors of convict prisons, 1918–1919 (1919), xxvii, cmd 374.

Report of the commissioners of prisons and the directors of convict prisons, 1919–20 (1920), xxiii, cmd 972.

Annual report of the commissioners of education in Ireland for 1919 (1920), xv, cmd 715.

Eighty-fifth report of the commissioners of national education in Ireland, 1918–19 (1920), cmd.1048.

Report upon the state of public health in the city of Dublin for the year 1919, by Sir Charles Cameron (Dublin, 1920).

Report upon the state of public health and the sanitary works performed in Dublin, 1911, by Sir Charles Cameron (Dublin, 1912).

Sixty-first annual report of the board of superintendence of the Dublin Hospitals for the year 1918–1919 (1919) cmd 480.

Contemporary journals

British Medical Journal, 1918–20.

Crofton, W.M, 'The influenza epidemic' in *Studies: Irish Quarterly Review of Letters, Philosophy and Science*, vii, no. 28 (1918), pp. 659–65.

Dublin Journal of Medical Science (January 1918 – June 1920).

Frost, W.H. and Sydenstricker, Edgar, 'Epidemic influenza in foreign countries' in *Public Health Reports* (1896–1970), xxxiv, no. 25 (Jun. 20, 1919), pp. 1361–76.

Hammond, J.A.R., Rolland W. and Shore, T.H.G., 'Purulent bronchitis', *Lancet*, ii (1917), p. 41.

Hennessy, Thomas, 'Medical reform for Ireland' in *The British Medical Journal*, i, no. 3039 (March 29, 1919).

Hennessy, Thomas, 'The report of the Irish Public Health Council', *British Medical Journal*, i, no. 3104 (26 June, 1920).

Levinson, A. 'Clinical observations on influenza with special reference to the blood and blood pressure', *The Journal of Infectious Diseases*, volume 25, no. 1, July, 1919, pp. 18–27.

MacNamara, D.W., 'Memories of 1918 and "the flu"', *Journal of Irish Medical Association*, xxxv, no. 208 (1954), 304–9.

Macnamara, D.W., 'The Mater – 1914–1919', *Journal of the Irish Medical Association*, xlix, no. 293 (November 1961).

Medical Press, 1918–20.

Peacocke, George, 'Influenza', *Dublin Journal of Medical Science*, 3rd series, no. 146 (1918), pp. 249–53.

Roesle, E., 'Classification of causes of deaths and death registration: principle and objects of the classification of the causes of death', *Journal of the American Statistical Association*, xxi, no. 154 (June, 1926), pp. 195–205.

Speares, John, 'Influenza', *Dublin Journal of Medical Science*, 3rd series, no. 146 (1918), pp. 253–258.

Thompson, W.J., 'Mortality from influenza in Ireland', *Dublin Journal of Medical Science*, 4th series (1920), pp. 174–86.

Thompson, W.J., 'Mortality from influenza in Ireland', *Journal of the Statistical and Social Inquiry Society of Ireland*, xiv (1919–20), pp. 1–14.

Newspapers

Carlow Nationalist, 1918–19.
Belfast Newsletter, 1918–19.
Dundalk Democrat and People's Journal, 1918–19.
Enniscorthy Echo, 1918–19.
Enniscorthy Guardian, 1918–19.
Evening Herald, 1918–19.
Irish Independent, 1918–19.
Irish Times, 1918–19.
Kildare Observer and Eastern Counties Advertiser, 1918–19.
Kilkenny People, 1918–19.
Leinster Leader, 1918–19.
Meath Chronicle, 1918–19.
Midland Tribune 1918–19.
Midland Reporter and Westmeath Nationalist, 1918–19.
Nationalist and Leinster Times, 1918–19.
Tipperary Star, 1919.
The People, 1918–19.
Weekly Irish Times, 1918–19.
Wicklow People, 1918–19.

Memoirs

Brennan, Robert, *Allegiance* (Dublin: Browne and Nolan, 1950).
Cameron, Sir Charles, *Autobiography of Sir Charles Cameron* (Dublin: Hodges Figgis, 1920).
Clarke, Kathleen, *Revolutionary Women: My Fight for Ireland's Freedom* (Dublin: O'Brien Press, 1997).
Gallagher, Frank, *The Four Glorious Years 1918–1921* (Tallaght: Blackwater Press, 2005; first edn 1953, under nom de plume David Hogan).
Graves, Robert, *Goodbye to All That*, rev. edn (London: Penguin, 1960).
O'Hegarty, P.S., *The Victory of Sinn Féin – How It Won It and How It Used It* (Dublin: UCD Press, 1998; first edn, 1924).
Price, Liam, ed., *Dr Dorothy Price: an Account of Twenty Years Fight Against Tuberculosis in Ireland*, priv. circ. (Oxford, 1957).
Robinson, Henry, *Memories Wise and Otherwise* (London: Cassell, 1923).
Robinson, Henry, *Further Memories of Irish Life* (London: H. Jenkins, 1924).

Specialist subjects

Adolphe Abrahams, 'Influenza: some clinical and therapeutic considerations', in F.G. Crookshank, *Influenza: Essays by Several Authors* (London: Heineman, 1922) pp. 314–50.

Crookshank, F. G., ed., *Influenza: Essays by Several Authors* (London: Heineman, 1922).

Hamer, W.H., 'The phases of influenza' in F.G. Crookshank, ed., *Influenza: Essays by Several Authors* (London: Heineman, 1922) pp. 102–27.

Jordan, E. O., *Epidemic Influenza: a Survey* (Chicago, IL: American Medical Association, 1927).

MacCallum, W.G. *A Text-Book of Pathology* (London: Saunders, 1918).

MacPherson, W.G, Horrocks, W.H., and Beveridge, W.W.O. *Medical Services Hygiene of the War*, from the series History of the Great War based on official documents (London: His Majesty's Stationery Office, 1923).

Mitchell, T.J., and Smith, G.M., *Medical Services – Casualties and Medical Statistics of the Great War*, from the series History of the Great War based on official documents (London: His Majesty's Stationery Office, 1931).

Jelliffe, Smith Ely, 'The nervous syndromes of influenza', in F.G. Crookshank, ed., *Influenza: Essays by Several Authors* (London: Heinemann, 1922), pp. 351–77.

White, W.H. *Materia Medica*, seventh edn. (London, 1902).

Secondary sources

Unpublished theses

Foley, Caitríona, 'The last Irish plague: the Great Flu in Ireland 1918–19' (PhD thesis, University College Dublin, 2009).

Johnson, N.P.A.S., 'Aspects of the historical geography of the 1918–1919' (PhD thesis, Cambridge), 2001.

Kidd, Cecil W., 'Epidemic influenza, an historical and clinical survey' (MD, Queen's University Belfast), 1933.

Marsh, Patricia, 'The effect of the 1918–19 influenza pandemic on Ulster' (PhD thesis, Queen's University Belfast), 2010.

Murphy, William, 'The Tower of Hunger: political imprisonment and the Irish 1910–1921' (PhD thesis, University College Dublin, 2006).

Tomkins, Sandra, 'Britain and the influenza pandemic of 1918–1919', PhD thesis, Cambridge, 1989.

Journals

Aronowitz, Robert, 'Lyme disease: The social construction of a new disease and its social consequences', *The Milbank Quarterly*, lxix, no. 1 (1991), pp. 79–112.

Beiner, Guy, and Bryson, Anna, 'Listening to the past and talking to each other: problems and possibilities facing oral history in Ireland', *Irish Economic and Social History*, xxx (2003), pp. 71–8.

Beiner, Guy, Marsh, Patricia, and Milne, Ida, 'Greatest killer of the twentieth century: the great flu in 1918–19', *History Ireland* (March–April 2009), pp. 40–3.

Brophy, Thomas J., 'On church grounds: political funerals and the contest to lead Catholic Ireland', *The Catholic Historical Review*, vol. 95, no. 3 (July 2009), pp. 491–514.

Colgan, John, and Cormack, David, 'Leixlip-Confey Gravestowns', *Journal of the County Kildare Archaelogical Society*, xix, part 3 (2004–5), p. 502.

Dunn, H.L., 'The evaluation of the effect upon mortality statistics of the selection of the primary cause of death', *Journal of the American Statistical Association*, vol. 31, no. 193 (March, 1936), pp. 113–23.

Engberg, Elisabeth, 'The invisible influenza: community response to pandemic influenza in rural northern Sweden 1918–20', *Vária Historia*, xlii, no. 25, 2009, pp. 429–56.

Froggatt, Peter, 'Sir William Wilde, 1815–1876: A centenary appreciation of Wilde's place in medicine', Proceedings of the Royal Irish Academy. Section C: *Archaeology, Celtic Studies, History, Linguistics, Literature,* vol. 77 (1977), pp. 261–78.

Mamelund, Svenn-Erik, 'A socially neutral disease? Individual social class, household wealth and mortality from Spanish influenza in two socially contrasting parishes in Kristiania 1918–19', *Social Science & Medicine*, lxii, no. 4 (2006), pp. 923–40.

Markel, Howard, Stern, Alexandra, and Cetron, Martin, 'Nonpharmaceutical interventions employed by major American cities during the 1918–1919 influenza pandemic', *Transactions of the American Clinical and Climatological Association*, no. 119 (2008), pp. 129–42.

Milne, Ida, 'The Big Flu in Wexford', *The Past: The Organ of the Uí Cinsealaigh Historical Society*, no. 27 (2006), pp. 50–5.

Mitka, Mike, '1918 Killer flu virus reconstructed, may help prevent future outbreaks', *Journal of the American Medical Association*, ccxciv, no. 19 (2005), pp. 2416–19.

Moore, George, 'Influenza and Parkinson's disease', *Public Health Reports* (*1974–*), pp. 79–80.

Morens, David, and Taubenberger, Jeffery, 'Understanding influenza backward', *Journal of the American Medical Association*, cccii, no. 6 (2009), pp. 679–80.

Mortimer, P.P., 'Was encephalitis lethargica a post-influenzal or some other phenomenon? Time to re-examine the problem', *Epidemiology and Infection*, xxxvii, no. 4 (April 2009), pp. 449–5.

Ó Bric, Deaglan, 'Pierce McCan MP. Part 1, 1882–1916' in *Tipperary Historical Journal*,(1988), pp. 121–32.

Oxford, J.S., Lambkin, R., Sefton, A., Daniels, R., Elliot, A., Brown, R., and Gill, D., 'A hypothesis: the conjunction of soldiers,gas, pigs, ducks, geese and horses in Northern France during the Great War provided the conditions for the emergence of the 'Spanish' influenza pandemic of 1918–1919', *Vaccine*, xxiii (2005), pp. 940–45.

Ryan, Desmond, 'The great influenza epidemic, 1918–1919', *Old Limerick Journal*, no. 33 (1996), pp. 50–1.

Smallman-Raynor, Matthew, Johnson, Niall, and Cliff, Andrew D., 'The spatial anatomy of an epidemic: Influenza in London and the County Boroughs of England and Wales, 1918–1919', *Transactions of the Institute of British Geographers*, new series, xxvii, no. 4 (2002), pp. 452–70.

Taubenberger J.K., and Morens, D.M., '1918 influenza: the mother of all pandemics', *Emerging Infectious Diseases*, xii, no. 1 (January 2006), pp. 15–22.

Ward, Alan, 'America and the Irish problem 1899–1921', in *Irish Historical Studies*, xvi, no. 61 (March 1968), pp. 64–90.

Books

Augusteijn, Joost, ed., *The Irish Revolution, 1913–1923* (Basingstoke: Palgrave, 2002).

Barrington, Ruth, *Health, Medicine and Politics in Ireland 1900–1970* (Dublin: Institute of Public Administration, 2000).

Barry, J.M., *The Great Influenza* (London: Penguin Books 2005).

Benjamin, B, *Elements of Vital Statistics* (London: Allen and Unwin, 1959).

Bergen Leo van, *Before My Helpless Sight: Suffering, Dying and Military Medicine on the Western Front, 1914–1918* (Farnham: Ashgate, 2009).

Berkow, Robert, ed., *Merck Manual of Diagnosis and Therapy* (Rahway, NJ: Merck Sharp & Dohme; 14th edn 1982).

Bornat, Joanna, 'Oral history as a social movement', in Robert Perks and Alastair Thomson, eds., *The Oral History Reader* (London: Routledge, 1998), pp. 189–205.

Caldwell Crosby, Molly, *Asleep: the Forgotten Epidemic that Remains One of Medicine's Greatest Mysteries*, electronic edn (New York: Berkley Books, 2010).

Campbell, F.J.M., *The Irish Establishment, 1879–1914* (Oxford: Oxford University Press, 2009.

Carroll, Lydia, *In the Fever King's Preserves: Sir Charles Cameron and the Dublin Slums* (Dublin: A & A Farmar, 2011).

Collier, Richard, *The Plague of the Spanish Lady* (London: Macmillan, 1974; paperback edn, 1996).

Colum, Padraic, *Arthur Griffith* (Dublin: Browne and Nolan, 1959).

Connolly, S.J., ed. *The Oxford Companion to Irish History* (Oxford: Oxford University Press, 1998).

Crosby, Alfred, *America's Forgotten Pandemic*, second edn (Cambridge: Cambridge University Press, 2003).

Crossman, Virginia, *Politics, Pauperism and Power in Late 19th Century Ireland* (Manchester: Manchester University Press, 2006).

Crossman, Virginia, and Lucey, Sean, eds, *Healthcare in Ireland and Britain 1850–1970: Voluntary, Regional and Comparative Perspectives* (London: Institute for Historical Research, 2015).

Daly, M.E., *Dublin the Deposed Capital: a Social And Economic History 1860–1914* (Cork: Cork University Press, 1984).

Daly, M.E., *The Buffer State –the historical roots of the Department of the Environment* (Dublin: Institute of Public Administration, 1997).

Echenberg. Myron, 'The dog that did not bark: memory and the 1918 influenza epidemic in Senegal', in Howard Phillips and David Killingray, eds, *The Spanish Influenza Pandemic of 1918–1919* (Abingdon: Routledge, 2003), pp. 230–8.

Echeverri, Beatriz, 'Spanish influenza seen from Spain', in Howard Phillips and David Killingray, eds, *The Spanish Influenza Pandemic of 1918–1919: New Perspectives* (Abingdon: Routledge, 2003) pp. 173–90.

Foley, Caitriona, *The Last Irish Plague* (Dublin: Irish Academic Press, 2011).

Foy, Michael, *Michael Collins's Intelligence War* (Stroud: Sutton, 2006).

Glandon, Virginia, *Arthur Griffith and the Advanced Nationalist Press: Ireland, 1900–1922* (New York: Peter Lang, 1985).

Hays, J.N., *The Burdens of Disease* (New Brunswick, NJ: Rutgers University Press, 2003).

Herring, D. Ann, and Sattenspiel, Lisa, 'Death in winter: Spanish flu in the Canadian Sub-arctic, in Howard Phillips and David Killingray, eds, *The Spanish Influenza Epidemic of 1918–19 – New Perspectives* (Abingdon: Routledge, 2003), pp. 156–72.

Herring, D. Ann, and Swedlund, Alan, eds, *Plagues and Epidemics Infected Spaces Past and Present* (Oxford: Berg, 2010).

Honigsbaum, Mark, *Living with Enza. The Forgotten Story of Britain and the Great Flu Pandemic of 1918* (Basingstoke: Palgrave, 2009).

Johnson, Niall, 'Influenza in Britain in 1918–19', in Howard Phillips and David Killingray, eds., *The Spanish Influenza Pandemic of 1918–1919* (Abingdon Routledge, 2003), pp. 132–55.

Johnson, Niall, *Britain and the 1918–19 Influenza Pandemic – a Dark Epilogue* (Abingdon: Routledge, 2006).

Jones, Greta, and Malcolm, Elizabeth, eds, *Medicine, Disease and the State in Ireland, 1650–1940* (Cork: Cork University Press, 1999).

Jones, Greta, 'The campaign against tuberculosis in Ireland, 1899–1914', in Greta Jones and Elizabeth Malcolm, eds, *Medicine, Disease and the State in Ireland, 1650–1940* (Cork: Cork University Press, 1999), pp. 158–76.

Kolata, Gina, *Flu: The Story of the Great Influenza Pandemic of 1918 and the Search for the Virus That Caused It* (New York: Farrar, Straus and Giroux, 1999).

Laffan, Michael, *The Resurrection of Ireland – the Sinn Féin Party, 1916–1923* (Cambridge: Cambridge University Press, 1999).

Lummis, Trevor, 'Structure and validity in oral evidence' in Robert Perks and Alistair Thomson, eds., *The Oral History Reader* (London: Routledge, 1998), pp. 273–83.

Martin, Peter, 'Ending the pauper taint: medical benefit and welfare reform in Northern Ireland, 1921–39', in Virginia Crossman and Peter Gray, eds, *Poverty and Welfare in Ireland 1838–1948* (Dublin: Irish Academic Press, 2013), pp. 223–36.

Mac Lellan, Anne, *Dorothy Stopford Price, Rebel Doctor* (Newbridge: Irish Academic Press, 2014).

Marsh, Patricia, 'The war and influenza: the impact of the First World War on the 1918–19 influenza pandemic in Ulster', in Ian Miller and David Durbin, eds, *Medicine, Health and Irish Experiences of Conflict, 1914–45* (Manchester: Manchester University Press, 2016).

McConville, Sean, *Irish Political Prisoners, 1848–1922* (Abingdon: Routledge, 2003).

McDowell, R.B., *Crisis and Decline: the Fate of the Southern Unionists* (Dublin: Lilliput Press, 1997).

McGarry, Fearghal, *The Rising – Ireland: Easter 1916* (Oxford: Oxford University Press, 2011).

McGuire, James, and Quinn, James, eds, *Dictionary of Irish Biography* (Cambridge: Cambridge University Press, 2009).

Miller, Ian, 'Pain trauma and memory in the Irish War of Independence', in Fionnuala Dillane, Naomi McAreavey and Emilie Pine, eds, *The Body in Pain in Irish Literature and Culture* (Basingstoke: Palgrave MacMillan, 2016), pp. 117–34.

Milne, Ida, 'Influenza: the Irish Local Government Board's last great crisis', in Virginia Crossman and Sean Lucey, eds, *Healthcare in Ireland and Britain 1850–1970: Voluntary, Regional and Comparative Perspectives.* (London: Institute for Historical Research, 2015), pp. 217–36.

Milne, Ida, 'Stacking the coffins: the 1918–19 influenza pandemic in Dublin', in Lisa Marie Griffith and Ciarán Wallace, eds, *Grave Matters: Death and Dying in Dublin, 1500 to the Present* (Dublin: Four Courts Press, 2016), pp. 61–76.

Milne Ida, 'Through the eyes of a child: childhood experience of the 1918–19 influenza pandemic', in Anne McLellan and Alice Mauger, eds, *Growing Pains: Childhood Illness in Ireland 1750–1950* (Dublin: Irish Academic Press, 2013), pp. 159–74.

Mitchell, B.R., *International Historical Statistics. Europe 1750–2000* (Basingstoke: Palgrave Macmillan, 2003).

Morrissey, Thomas J., *Laurence O'Neill (1864–1943): Patriot and Man of Peace* (Dublin: Four Courts Press, 2014).

Müller, Jürgen, 'Bibliography' in Howard Phillips and David Killingray, eds., *The Spanish Influenza Pandemic of 1918–19* (Abingdon: Routledge, 2003).

Murphy, William, *Political Imprisonment and the Irish* (Oxford: Oxford University Press, 2014).

Novick, Ben, 'Propaganda I: Advanced nationalist propaganda and moralistic revolution, 1914–1918', in Joost Augusteijn, ed., *The Irish Revolution, 1913–1923* (Basingstoke: Palgrave, 2002), pp. 34–52.

O'Brien, Gerard, 'State intervention and medical relief of the poor' in Greta Jones and Elizabeth Malcolm, eds., Medicine, *Disease and the State in Ireland, 1650–1940* (Cork: Cork University Press, 1999), pp. 195–207.

Ó Brolcháin, Honor, *All in the Blood* (Dublin: A & A Farmar, 2006).

O'Connor, Emmet, *A Labour History of Ireland, 1824–1960* (Dublin: University College Dublin Press, 2011).

Ó hÓgartaigh, Margaret, *Kathleen Lynn – Irishwoman, Patriot, Doctor* (Dublin: Irish Academic Press, 2006).

Olson, Kent, ed., *Poisoning and Drug Overdose* (London: Prentice-Hall, 1990).

Perks, Robert, and Thomson, Alistair, eds, *The Oral History Reader* (London: Routledge, 1998).

Phillip, Howard, *Black October: The Impact of the Spanish Influenza Epidemic of 1918 on South Africa* (Pretoria: Govt. Printer, 1990).

Phillips, Howard, and Killingray, David, eds, *The Spanish Influenza Pandemic of 1918–1919* (Abingdon: Routledge, 2003).

Porter, Katharine Anne, *Pale Horse, Pale Rider* (Orlando, FL: Harcourt Brace, 1939).

Porter, Roy, *The Greatest Benefit to Mankind*, paperback edn (London: Fontana Press, 1999).

Price, Frederick, ed., *A Textbook of the Practice of Medicine*, seventh edn (Oxford: Oxford University Press, 1947).

Price, Liam, ed., *Dr Dorothy Price, an Account of Twenty Years Fight Against Tuberculosis in Ireland*, priv. circ. (Oxford, 1957).

Ramona, Radula, 'The Bombay experience', in Phillips, Howard and Killingray, David, eds, *The Spanish Influenza Pandemic of 1918–1919* (Abingdon: Routledge, 2003), pp. 86–98.

Ranger, Terence, and Slack, Paul, eds, *Epidemics and Ideas: Essays on the Historical Perception of Pestilence* (Cambridge: Cambridge University Press, 1992).

Rice, Geoffrey, *Black November: The 1918 Influenza Pandemic in New Zealand.* (Christchurch, NZ: Canterbury University Press, 2005).

Robins, Joseph, *Custom House People* (Dublin: Dublin Institute of Public Administration, 1993).

Roche, Desmond, *Local Government*, second edn (Dublin: Institute of Public Administration, 1963).

Rosenberg, Charles, *Explaining Epidemics and Other Studies in the History of Medicine* (Cambridge: Cambridge University Press, 1999).

Silverstein, Arthur, *Pure Politics and Impure Science: the Swine Flu Affair* (Baltimore, MD: Johns Hopkins University Press, 1981).

Taubenberger, Jeffery, 'Genetic characterisation of the 1918 "Spanish" influenza virus', in Howard Phillips and David Killingray, eds, *The Spanish Influenza Pandemic of 1918–1919* (Abingdon: Routledge, 2003).

Thompson, Paul, *The Voice of the Past – Oral History* (Oxford: Oxford University Press, 2000).

White, W.H., *Materia Medica*, seventh edn (London, 1902).

Winter, Jay, and Roberts, J.L., eds, *Capital Cities at War – Paris, London, Berlin 1914–1919* (Cambridge: Cambridge University Press, 1997).

Zinsser, Hans, *Rats, Lice and History* (Boston, MA: Little, Brown, 1935).

Television programmes
Outbreak, produced by Janet Gallagher, RTE 1, 2 June, 2009.
Aicid, produced by Mary Jones, TG4 and BBC Northern Ireland, November 2008, 1 June 2009.

Websites
Centers for Disease Control, www/cdc/gov/flu 7 May 2009.
CDC, 'Pandemic Flu Storybook', 2008. www.cdc.gov/about/panflu/ 7 May 2009.
Hall, William, 'Report on pandemic preparedness, 2007' in www.ucd.ie/news/jan07/011907_pandemic_report.htm 23 March 2007.
Health Protection Surveillance Centre, www.hpsc.ie/ 7 May 2009.
Health Services Executive, www.hse.ie 7 May 2009.
National Disease Surveillance Centre. www.ndsc.ie/Disease Topics A-Z/InfluenzaFlu/Influenza 8 June 2005.

Pandemic Influenza Expert Group, Modelling impact of pandemic influenza: interim report on use of empirical model in Ireland. See www.ndsc. ie/hpsc/A-Z/EmergencyPlanning/AvianPandemicInfluenzaPreparedne ssforIreland/Suplement3toChapter3/File220.en.pdf December 2006, 10 October 2010.

World Health Organization, www.who.int/csr/disease/influenza/ pandemic10things/en/ 5 October 2010.

World Health Organization. www.who.int/classifications/icd/en/ HistoryOfICD.pdf 9 June 2005.

Conference papers

Engberg, Elisabeth, 'Caring for the fatherless: epidemic influenza and family dissolution in Sweden, 1920', paper presented to the ESSHC conference, Ghent, April 2010.

Geary, Laurence, 'Medicine and the State: the Poor Law medical service in Ireland, 1851–1921' in the Mackey Lecture series, National Library of Ireland, February 2010.

Marsh, Patricia, '"Sleepy sickness spread": encephalitis lethargica in Belfast', paper presented at Society for the Social History of Medicine conference, Canterbury, July 2016.

Oeppen, Jim, Garcia Ferrero, Sara and Ramiro Fariñas, Diego, 'Estimating reproductive numbers for the 1889–90 and 1918–20 influenza pandemic in Madrid', paper presented to the European Social Science History Conference, Ghent, April 2010.

Oxford, John, 'Epidemics past present and future', public lecture in the Paccar Theatre, The Science Gallery, Trinity College, Dublin, May 2010.

Index